T0246619

THE ART OF ANATOMY
IN MEDIEVAL EUROPE

Covering one of the most fascinating yet misunderstood periods in history, the MEDIEVAL LIVES series presents medieval people, concepts and events, drawing on political and social history, philosophy, material culture (art, architecture and archaeology) and the history of science. These books are global and wide-ranging in scope, encompassing both Western and non-Western subjects, and span the fifth to the fifteenth centuries, tracing significant developments from the collapse of the Roman Empire onwards.

SERIES EDITOR: Deirdre Jackson

Albertus Magnus and the World of Nature *Irven M. Resnick and Kenneth F. Kitchell Jr*

Alle Thyng Hath Tyme: Time and Medieval Life *Gillian Adler and Paul Strohm*

Andrey Rublev: The Artist and His World *Robin Milner-Gulland*

The Art of Anatomy in Medieval Europe *Taylor McCall*

Christine de Pizan: Life, Work, Legacy *Charlotte Cooper-Davis*

Margery Kempe: A Mixed Life *Anthony Bale*

THE ART OF ANATOMY IN MEDIEVAL EUROPE

TAYLOR McCALL

REAKTION BOOKS

For J.R.M. I and II

Published by Reaktion Books Ltd
Unit 32, Waterside
44–48 Wharf Road
London N1 7UX, UK
www.reaktionbooks.co.uk

First published 2023
Copyright © Taylor McCall 2023

Printed and bound in India by Replika Press Pvt. Ltd

A catalogue record for this book is available from the British Library

ISBN 978 1 78914 681 3

CONTENTS

Introduction   7

PART I: ANATOMY AND COSMOS

1 Spiritual Anatomy and the Monastery   32

2 Blood and Stars: Anatomical Astrology   63

PART II: ANATOMY AND SURGERY

3 Cutting Cadavers: Surgeons, Anatomy and
  the Establishment of Human Dissection   83

4 Fourteenth-Century Anatomical Images,
  Latin West and Islamic Middle East   106

PART III: ANATOMY AND ARTISTS

5 Decorating the Text: Professional Artists
  and the Anatomical Page   126

6 The Anatomy of a Scene: Dissection in
  Manuscript and Print, c. 1400–1540   157

Conclusion   177

REFERENCES   181
SELECT BIBLIOGRAPHY   209
ACKNOWLEDGEMENTS   215
PHOTO ACKNOWLEDGEMENTS   217
INDEX OF MANUSCRIPTS CITED   219
GENERAL INDEX   221

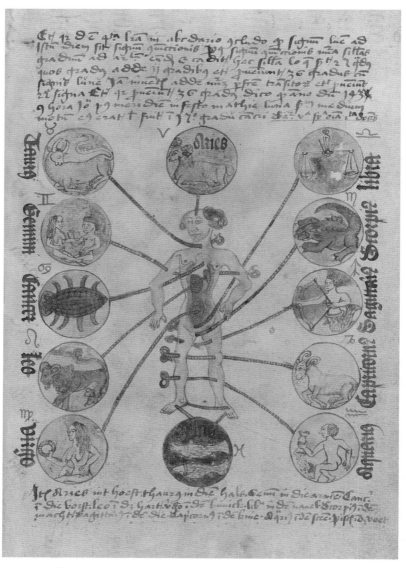

1 Zodiac anatomical figure, from Heymandus de Veteri Busco,
Ars computistica (1488).

Introduction

What expectations do we bring with us when looking at diagrams of human anatomy? Most might say they would hope these types of images – like other scientific graphics – present impartial information, free from ideological biases: the make-up of the body as it is. But we also understand that diagrams are not copies of reality. They seek to communicate information in as easy a manner as possible, often at the expense of visual fact, not limited by what we can see in real life: to depict the lungs, the ribs might be omitted for a clearer view; to demonstrate insemination, the entire process may appear in step-by-step phases within the same image of the female reproductive system. Descriptive captions are often crucial superimpositions to explain what is being represented, and these, of course, cannot be found organically. Furthermore, the information they communicate is based on someone's opinion of what is most important, which might differ from another's.

Just as modern anatomical diagrams are subjective, so too were medieval ones, created to express different viewpoints of or information about the body.[1] They were not intended to communicate a unified, empirical 'knowledge' of the make-up or processes of the interior. In addition, emphasis in medieval anatomical learning was on physiological function rather than the organization of the parts within the interior space of the body, as is often the emphasis in modern-day anatomy.[2] Medieval anatomical images

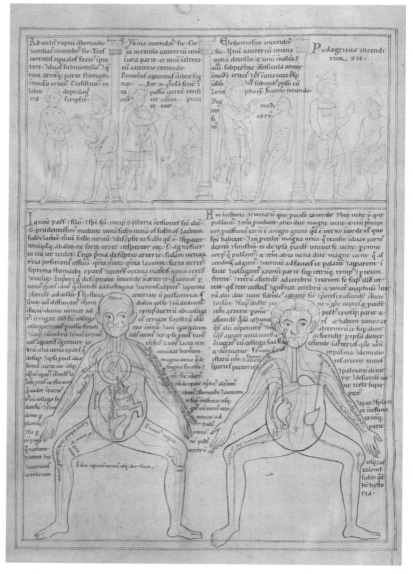

2, 3 The Five-Figure Series (above: cautery scenes atop diagrams of veins and arteries; opposite: bones, nerves and muscles), from *Glossarium Salomonis* (c. 1165).

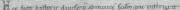

Hec sunt hystorie diuisorum abinuicem sedin que instruunt.

ea faber. e. plasmate eoru induidritq; ea neruu. earo et ner
ut estringunt unu alteru. Inutriu boz ossuu e calsti. et e po
sitio et rotunda. subqua cerebru habitat. Ipq; ut decurrit
medulla ispondulo neruel. et colligant iuce eu illo. et eum
osse barbe. et ipse ascendunt. Lacrime. uocant. musculi. et
eex gaudin. iirinsecus. ac. minutissima ossa imodu
sisam. Nasus aut pcedit abintio ossis qd e ime
dio oculoz. et e cartillagi. igene eu mandi
bule. et ehina eoz. eninguiz. tur ossi radicel auriuz.
et uocantur seuta. et i ipsis sunt dentes et nu
merus eoz omnium.

Hee e hystoria neruoru qui si ligamina corporis et ossuu
et uenaru et locutoru qui corpore o sic condidit et plasma
uit ea sapientissimus dns. Principio pedum duo magni
neruu pimedulla ispondyloz. qui retra o. et cooperiunt eos
eu colliega suo. et eltrin gunt. et eternuat. ad
nec pueniant adcerru em. Inde sumitates
neruoru ilstog. et exra q; parte ascendunt
sup caput. et iucem colligant. ibi induo
bus modis rotundus. et iteriu pcedit. decerebro
et nerual et descendit mammeriore parte capu
et frontis. et ubi ap paret diuiditur
indue. qui cu ligantur in
duo oculos.
ritim diut si puent
uni ul uni ocu
lo. ualt alteri
et mini triaq;
illa lum i neruo
ius. he

ossa gutturis sunt sponda
li. et et ibi aliud osquod
sudatur. Hongema. et
iterum ossa oculoruz
sunt posita. facie ad fari
em. et sunt septem et
de ipsis fiunt coste. Coste
uero laterir deerteri complere
et iparte sinistra est minu costa
una imasculo. Ifemina s eplere. Reliq s hystorie

ris est pforat. iduo mag
nneru descendunt imaxillas. Ire uer
tumur ad supiore neruu capitis. et proce
dit ner uus ad cap. qse e par primo et det
cendit in pecruus. Icolligant ille. et deri uatur
quousq; uadit. et reuis par descendir i trin
secus. et uenas. parte usq; ad ambas
palmas. sedm quod uj d e s.

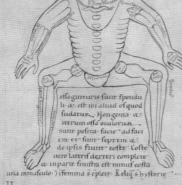

Hee s hystoria lacerruz. qs sec dns ut uacui replea. icuingat
qd separat e. Is et modis. Ilmo modo ut caro. alia neq; ut caro. ne
q; ut cib s medul. Tertius dissimili apimo q. asedo. et
uocat musculi. Ipuplui pot mouere corp us. et
tere motione sedin uo bia ut apiam. Iioinm
marilla. Iadiunat os. Ili di. Irim duo pare musei
morione oris fiunt. iphan de gluriar. Iponar. et de
lus s. Iad inuat of ut apa ioim motione sua
ponar spm. Iduo hoz. deorsu et ro
et adiuuat euce acur. Iin
Ihu ipse here s et con
runda. Iursu iuce iuce
iue euune parte
inguiri
muriq;
cerruu rubii
iuetre st adde roe
tione cibuz merigen
do et decli nibus
sunt adiu Ihu q
s iuearis ea in
et digestione ad iuuant
nando ut iterum hii qui ima
uant ea imom morione sua
et eruribus et talo adiuuant
omm motione s y a.

Mense ianuario reponeus. Mense febr agrimonia. et
apii sem. Mense martio ruta. Ielutisco. Mense aprili be
tonica. Ipibinella. Mense maio absinthiu Ihenseili sem
Mense iunio. saluie flores. Isauina. Mense iulio flo
res deapio Iuua. Mense augusti puleiu. Mense septebri
cotto Igramia attee. Mense octob. gariofolo et piper
Mense nouemb cinamo. Mense decembri spico. Mense ma
io gamandria et humore frangendu. Mense iunio. iris
lingua. apiu. pip. ad oleari stringendu. ut solutione
faciend. Mense iulio. cardone eu qinq; grams pipi Mse
augusto. saluie. puleiu. actione eu pip. Mense septebri
betonica eu pip. Mense octob. sauina eu sale. Mse
nouemb. Igramina. ysopo et saureia. pstomacho. Men
se ian. februario. sarmina eu sale. Mense mar. puleio
o adstomacho calefaciendu. Mense apli renu purum
qinq; die monato bibar. Posta ipse anno iiisebre i
timet cadere. Mense mar. puleiu bibar dulcia uta
Iradicei efcetas aspario eu sanguine n minuat
nec solutione accipiat qa ipsa solutio frigora generat
Mense apli sanguine minuere solutione accipe recen
tes carnel n manduca. sanguine irricancai minu
ere. calidu utere. stomachu purgare. ungentis cald
tiea utere. si sie fuir om ii ibra sanare. Mense maio
calidu bibar. calidu usere cap purgare. qa caldu iialore pre
cordi ponit. Vena capitis medii hoc. Iuena epariea solum
one. bibere. prurigine mundare. urina purgare. cibu fri
gidare. Mi. iunio. cottidie ieiui calsce de aqua bibar. et cer
uisia bibar. Ibutisei. Ieruuai edar. et calidu bibar. Mi. iulio.

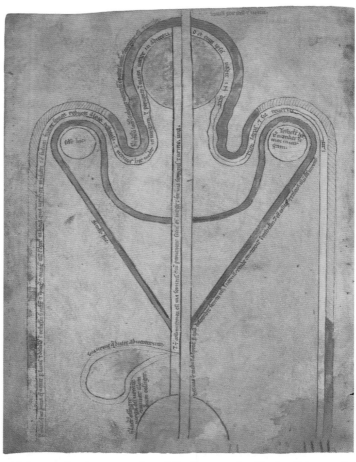

4 Male reproductive system, from *Miscellanea medica* [England] (c. 1200).

range from neat, simplified full-body figures dedicated to a single 'system' (the bones, for instance; illus. 3) to abstracted internal views of individual organs (illus. 4, 5), to scenes of a cadaveric dissection (illus. 6). Some imaginative compositions depict dissected bodies, viscera exposed, interacting spryly with their anatomists (illus. 7). Others underline the perceived connections between the parts of the body and the universe, the organs superimposed with or linked to zodiac symbols (illus. 1). Created

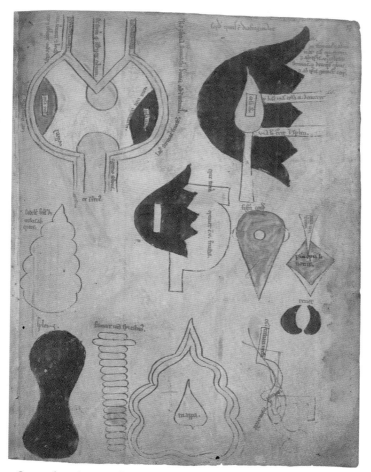

5 Stomach and internal organs, from *Miscellanea medica* [England]
(*c.* 1200).

between approximately 1150 and 1500, these diverse illustrative
modes speak to the different motivations and priorities of the
hands that drew them. For instance, monks might have drawn
diagrams that helped them to better understand the relationship
between the body and the heavens in accordance with God's
divine design; surgeons might have consulted them to learn the
connections between the organs to accurately perform their

procedures; professional manuscript artists might have painted them to signpost the contents of different chapters in a medical text.

Although varied, medieval anatomical images were relatively rare, and this combination of variety and paucity has meant they have mostly been included in broader surveys of scientific or medical images, or as historical background to studies on the better-known advancements made in early modern and Renaissance anatomy, but have not been the focus of a dedicated study in modern scholarship.[3] Part of this lacuna stems from a lack of consensus over what exactly constitutes an anatomical diagram. A recent catalogue of global anatomical images from prehistory to the present day demonstrates just how difficult the word 'anatomy' is to delineate, and the editors ultimately chose to include representations of the interior and exterior of the body across genres and media, not restricted to those created for medical purposes.[4] Over the past thirty years, scholars have increasingly investigated the connection between bodies in medieval art and their relationship to the medieval person's experience, and anatomical images have either been avoided entirely or mentioned in passing, perhaps because they resist traditional academic classifications, sitting between art history and medical history. Many of these contributions have focused on themes that touch on anatomical topics, especially the gendered body: specifically, the manipulation of the female form, the role of the sexes in reproduction and generation, and queer and transgender experiences and sexuality.[5]

By situating anatomical diagrams as the central focus, this book seeks to build and expand on these topics, exposing the unique perspective these images can shed on many contemporary debates. By concentrating on diagrams of bodies and organs created in learned anatomical contexts – representations of the interior found in manuscripts and printed works produced in or

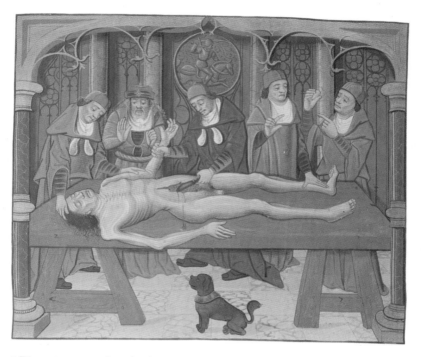

6 Dissection scene, from book v of Bartholomew the Englishman,
Livre des propriétés des choses (c. 1475–1500).

for educated medical circles, in which the priority was the depiction of the body for didactic or practical purposes relating to
treatment – we are best able to trace the different ways in which
particular makers approached the human body in the context of
the development of anatomy as a field of knowledge. While we
will touch upon exposed interiors in non-educational contexts,
the focus will be on anatomical images made to illustrate medical texts. The earliest anatomical images appeared in the twelfth
century, in monastic and then early university settings; at the start
of the fourteenth century, we have the first evidence of human
dissection since the short-lived experimentations in Hellenistic
Greece over a thousand years before. The fifteenth century saw
the establishment of Western printing and the spread of academic

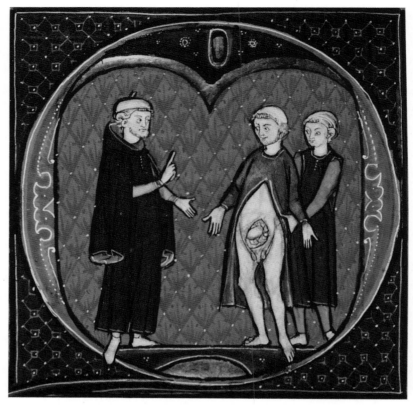

7 Historiated initial featuring a physician (Avicenna?) gesturing
to a dissected figure, from Avicenna, *Canon* (*c.* 1260).

cadaveric dissections in universities. The effects of these major
events on the field of anatomy can be charted through analysis
of the illustrations crafted to elucidate textual descriptions.

Simply put, this book's focus will be on the makers who
drew the interior in order to explain an overarching idea about
the functioning of the physical body, be that in a medical, cosmological or moralistic sense. I am by no means proposing an
exclusive definition of anatomy that dismisses representations
of decomposing bodies, skeletons and the human figure in general outside the realm of learned anatomy. Nor am I advocating

for the disregard of anatomical images that do not appear with related texts.[6] Rather, the intent is to position this study as one that engages foremost with shifting theories surrounding the physical composition and processes of the body, and how those ideas were translated into a visual language. This includes representations of anatomy's 'sister' practice, autopsy, as a practical application of surgery and dissection that was accepted in religious circles as a means for discovering evidence of divine favour in holy bodies, and as a public health service necessary for legal and civic investigations into poisonings, deliberate and accidental.

The images presented here have been divided into three broadly conceived thematic sections: Anatomy and Cosmos, Anatomy and Surgery and Anatomy and Artists. These are not meant to be hard-and-fast dividers, as there are many overlaps between the images sorted into these spheres. By delving into the similarities and contrasts between their graphic priorities, this book will highlight the role of anatomical images in medical learning and the richly creative ways in which medieval artists and scientists, united by a shared desire to illuminate the interior, worked.

Background: The Origins of Anatomical Learning in the West

Western European medieval anatomy can be simplistically explained as a synthesis: the opinions of the ancient medical authorities – Hippocrates (fifth and fourth centuries BCE), Aristotle (384–322 BCE) and Galen of Pergamum (129–c. 216 CE) chief among them – preserved, abridged and enhanced by Middle Eastern authors, and subsequently translated into Latin. Added to this core corpus over the period in focus here (roughly, 1100–1500) was a steady trickle of newly discovered works by classical authors as well as original texts by medieval scholars. What follows is a summary of the foundation upon which Western medieval anatomy was built.

The earliest medical treatises, those associated with the mythical Hippocrates, indicate that seeing and mapping the human interior was secondary in importance to understanding the body's physiological processes in a more theoretical manner.[7] The Hippocratic oeuvre contains neither references to human dissection nor any accompanying images, and stresses the significance of understanding the diverse ways in which the four humours – black bile, red bile, blood and phlegm – affected various organs and body parts. A successful remedy for an illness or injury could only be prescribed with accurate knowledge of these concepts.

Like the Hippocratic corpus, Aristotle's priority was to understand the operation of various body parts and how they acted together to achieve a specific overall function. In other words, he focused on an understanding of causes, rather than anatomical forms. Aristotle's emphasis on teleology and envisioning the body as a series of discrete parts would be fundamental in establishing influential later approaches – for example, that of Galen – as well as profoundly impacting the study of anatomy well beyond the Renaissance. There is no evidence Aristotle performed human dissections; however, his texts on animals include detailed observations of the internal organs, which could have reasonably been achieved through dissection, and his zoological works make several comparisons between animal and human bodily processes.[8] He also occasionally cites accompanying images in his works.[9] While these are now lost, they are among the earliest explicit references to anatomical figures.

The only recorded instances of scientific human dissection before the practice was re-established in the fourteenth century by medieval surgeons were performed by Greek physicians

Herophilus and Erasistratus in Alexandria in the first half of the third century BCE.[10] Such experiments indicate a desire to understand the secrets of the interior by going beyond the visible exterior, yet they had no evident precedent and were apparently discontinued after their deaths, and there are no visual records of their efforts.

Approximately four centuries after Herophilus and Erasisratus, the Greek physician Galen left his indelible mark on the field of anatomical exploration.[11] Galen believed one could not adequately practice medicine without a firm knowledge of anatomy. Galen did not dissect human cadavers, although his medieval followers believed he did based on his detailed descriptions of anatomy and praise of dissection as integral to medical practice. However, he did conduct numerous public dissections of animals believed to have similar organs to humans, such as pigs and apes, and continually asserted the importance of anatomical understanding in his writings. He also performed surgical procedures and exhorted his readers to mimic his experiments and dissections to witness his discoveries at first hand. The scope of Galen's influence is evidenced by the hundreds of works written by him, claiming to be penned by him or somehow connected to him from both the East and the West in the 1,300 years after his death.

Most of the medical learning of the West was formed by the scholars and writers of the Middle East, especially those working in modern-day Iraq and Iran.[12] The works of classical authorities were preserved in libraries in Alexandria and Byzantium and brought to the courts of the Islamic Middle East beginning in the eighth and ninth centuries.[13] Broadly, the medical learning translated to Arabic between circa 700 and circa 1100 CE conformed to the teachings of Galen. His writings were considered too wordy and complicated and were edited and consolidated into encyclopaedic format, the most important of which were written by Abū Bakr Muḥammad ibn Zakariyyā al-Rāzī (known by his Latinized name as Rhazes, 854–925), 'Ali ibn al-'Abbas al-Majusi (Haly Abbas, d. 994), Ibn Sina (Avicenna, c. 980–1037), Abu al-Qasim Khalaf ibn al-'Abbas al-Zahrawi (Albucasis, *fl.* 912–61) and Abū l-Walīd Muḥammad ibn 'Aḥmad ibn Rušd (Averroes, 1126–1198). Despite the emphasis on encyclopaedic consolidation, there were many original contributions to anatomical knowledge made by medieval Middle Eastern physicians. Among the most influential was the *Kitāb al-Manāẓir* (Book of Optics), written in the early eleventh century by the Iraqi physician Ḥasan Ibn al-Haytham (Latinized as Alhazen or Alhacen,

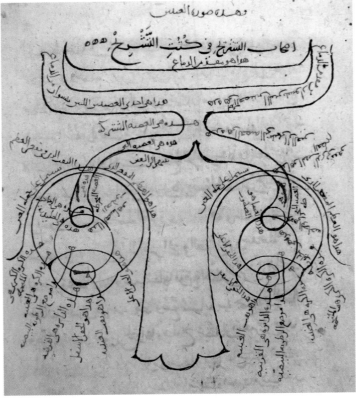

8 Brain and ocular system, from Ibn al-Haytham, *Kitāb al-Manāẓir* (1083; 15 Jumādā 1 476).

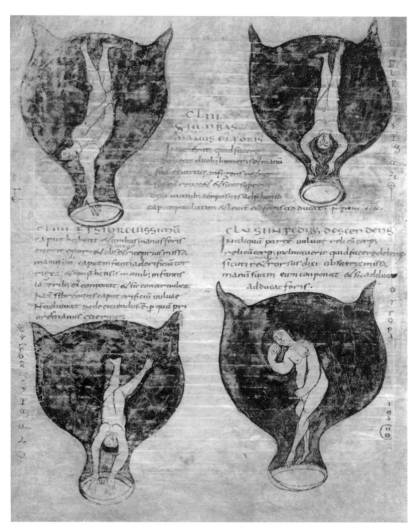

9 Foetal positions in the womb, from Muscio, *Gynaecia* (9th century).

c. 965–c. 1040).[14] Contrary to popular opinion, there was no religious ban on representing the body in medieval Islamic medical works.[15] Most medical compendia produced by Islamic physicians and authors have sections on anatomy, and some contain schematic diagrams, particularly of the cranial sutures and the eyeball, of which there is a diagram preserved in a copy made a few decades after the completion of the original *Kitāb al-Manāẓir* (illus. 8).[16]

Such medical and anatomical illustrations, however, were a rarity in Middle Eastern, Byzantine and European traditions in general. As one recent exploration of Western medical manuscripts made during the 'long' twelfth century (1095–1229) has proven, the few medical images dating from that period were copies of older graphic traditions, preserved in monastic manuscripts usually alongside other miscellaneous medical texts, and not newly created iconographies.[17] The most popular medical images before 1100 were images of flora and fauna associated with herbals, texts discussing the medical properties of plants, for which the earliest surviving codex example dates to the sixth century.[18] Depictions of cautery, the therapeutic burning of the body with strategically placed hot irons to drain the body of bad humours, appear in manuscripts as early as the tenth century (see illus. 2 at top left).[19] The only other type of pre-twelfth-century medical imagery is tangentially anatomical: drawings of the positions of foetuses in the womb that circulated with the treatise *Gynaecia* attributed to Muscio.[20] The oldest manuscript containing these images dates to the ninth century (illus. 9), the tiny homunculi arranged acrobatically within the round, red interiors of the bicornate uterus.

Emergence of a Medieval Anatomical Tradition

The earliest surviving Western medieval anatomical diagrams were drawn in the Bavarian monastery of Prüfening around 1165 as part of a series of images encouraging a reader to meditate on the relationship between the body and the divine (see illus. 2, 3). These five full-body figures, each representing a different system (veins, arteries, bones, nerves and muscles), appear a number of

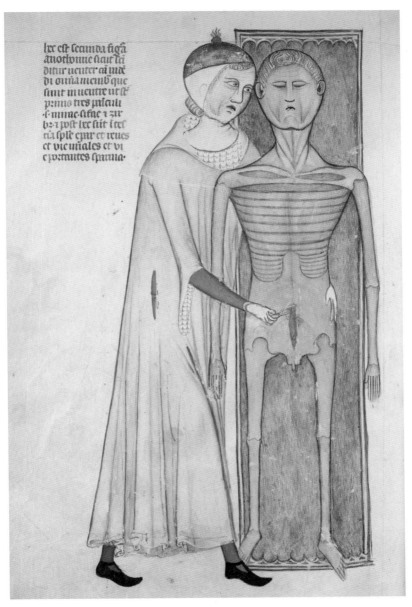

10 *Figura 2*: Guido of Vigevano dissecting a cadaver, from Guido of Vigevano, *Anatomia Philippi septimi* (1345).

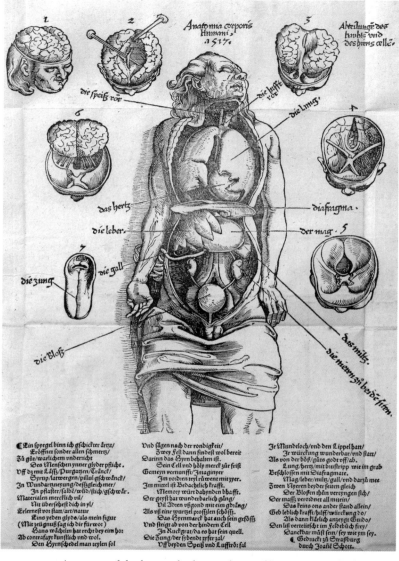

11 Anatomy of the human body, woodcut in Hans von Gersdorff, *Feldtbüch der Wundartzney* (1528), originally published in Wendelin Hock, *Ein contrafact Anatomy der inneren Glyderen des Menschen* . . . (1517).

times across Europe over the next three hundred years in both medical and religious manuscripts, evolving to fit shifting aesthetic notions of manuscript imagery in general and anatomical drawings in particular, and – in keeping with the scholarship on twelfth-century medical images – were most likely descended from a late antique tradition. In the early fourteenth century, educated surgeons created new visual accompaniments to their original anatomical manuals (illus. 10) for the first time. As the practice of human dissection increased in the years before the dawn of the sixteenth century, Europe's earliest printers included anatomical images as visual aids that both clung to older traditions and became progressively more detailed (illus. 11). At the same time, late medieval and early modern artists began to work with anatomists in order to improve their own understanding of and ability to depict the human form, beginning a collaboration that would see the elevation of anatomical diagrams to fine art, as in Leonardo da Vinci's (1452–1519) work (illus. 13).

The identities of the majority of the creators of medieval anatomical images are unknown monks, workshop illustrators and students who drew them for their own diverse purposes. Many of the images are workaday, unadorned and abstruse, which – coupled with the anonymity of their makers – accounts for a general lack of interest in them by the first several generations of medieval art historians. In addition, while the value of these images to different types of makers was myriad, the makers themselves were overwhelmingly uniform in terms of demographics. With very few exceptions, the world of European learned anatomy was made up of Christian, white males writing and learning in Latin. Although enclosed communities of religious women have existed for as long as male communities, we have no indication that women studied, copied or produced anatomical images inside monastic settings or out, and so they are absent from this study as makers.[21] Jewish practitioners were also instrumental in

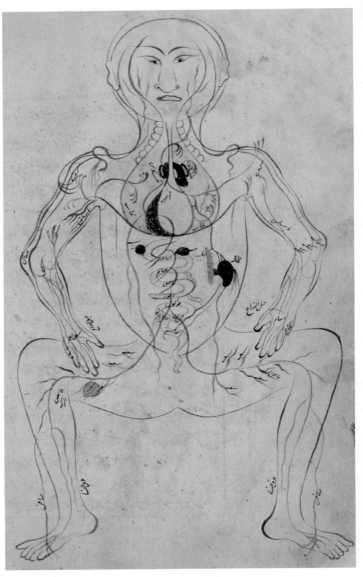

12 Veins, from Manṣūr ibn Ilyās, *Tashrīḥ-i Manṣūr-i* (1488).

13 Leonardo da Vinci, 'The cardiovascular system and principal organs of a woman', *c.* 1509–10, black and red chalk, pen and ink, and yellow wash on paper.

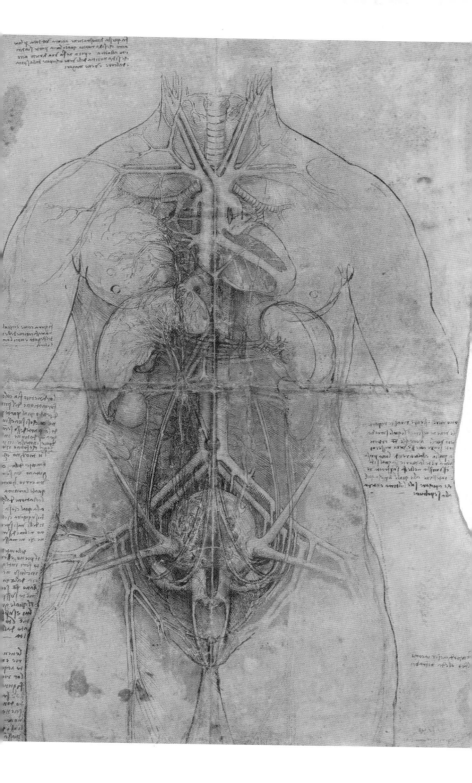

the growth of medical knowledge in the Middle Ages, but – to my knowledge – there are no Jewish authors or Hebrew texts associated with anatomical images.[22] Thus the vast majority of bodies portrayed in this book are white and male, the 'ideal' body.[23] A notable exception is the appearance of anatomical images in the Middle Eastern tradition in the later Middle Ages, featuring non-white bodies (illus. 12).[24] Women were considered to be deformed men, valued mostly for their role in reproduction;[25] as such, most female anatomical bodies are marked by the uterus and little else (illus. 14). Original owners of the manuscripts into which many of these images and texts were copied are often unidentified, but we can determine general priorities and attitudes based on contextual clues.

The diagrams explored here will be considered as both reflections of the medieval perception of the body within medicine and anatomy and as 'art' objects – products of careful design, meant to impact a viewer. For an educated medical student or practitioner, the images clarified the physiological theories of Galen, medicine's equivalent of a Church Father. For a religious viewer, the images could serve as reminders of the body's connection with both the larger cosmic universe and as a link with Christ, who suffered in the same flesh.

Investigating Interiors

I have organized this book around the people who made and used these images: monks, university anatomists, professional physicians, professional artists and artist-anatomists. These are broad categories that are not meant to be mutually exclusive, but rather to serve as a framework for considering the myriad ways in which anatomical images were created and understood. Although every effort has been made to discuss the full range of medieval anatomical images, this is not an exhaustive survey.

Part One, 'Anatomy and Cosmos', explores the inclusion of human anatomy in religious contexts. Chapter One examines both the role of monasteries in the story of anatomical learning, and enclosed monks as copiers, translators, artists and healers. Monasteries in the West inherited and preserved the writings of antiquity, and the monastic life valued the acts of copying and writing as one of a monk's sacred duties to glorify God. Medical treatises were copied, circulated as practical tools to maintain the health of a monastic community and the laypeople in the surrounding areas, and consulted as an additional way to understand the body as a microcosm of the universe. We see the inclusion of anatomical and medical materials and images in otherwise strictly religious books. Chapter Two progresses this discussion by exploring the widespread use of anatomical imagery in diagrams associated with medical astrology (known as melothesia) in the later Middle Ages. These images visually spell out the perceived links between the planets and zodiac and the parts of the body, appearing in religious and scientific manuscripts alike. They remained popular well into the early modern period.

Part Two, 'Anatomy and Surgery', delves into the role of anatomical imagery within the realm of university medical teaching and practice. The establishment of universities as places of learning outside monasteries – albeit initially primarily comprised of monks and other clerics – paved the way for the professionalization of medicine. Chapter Three will consider the fight for the recognition of surgery as a university-worthy discipline rather than simply a manual craft, and the subsequent elevation of anatomy as an important aspect of surgical study by the earliest generations of educated surgeons. Italian surgeons, most notably Mondino dei Liuzzi (c. 1265–1326), were the first known individuals to perform human dissections in the context of scientific exploration since Herophilus and Erasistratus. Other surgeons, especially Henry of Mondeville (c. 1260–1320) and Guido of

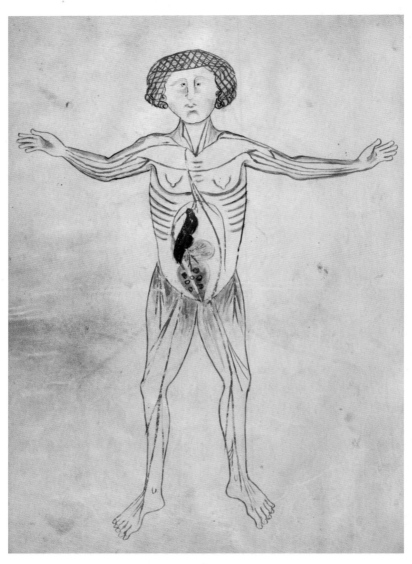

14 Anatomy of a woman, from *Miscellanea medica* [southern France] (*c.* 1300).

Vigevano (*c.* 1280–*c.* 1349), recognized the benefit of including images to demonstrate anatomical principles in their own original texts. Chapter Four explores Guido's unique diagrams, in which he depicts himself dissecting corpses – the first to do so, and some two hundred years before Andreas Vesalius (1514–1564) would famously do the same. Chapter Four also focuses on the non-Western diagrams accompanying Mansūr ibn Muḥammad ibn Amād ibn Yūsuf ibn Ilyās's (*fl.* 1380–1420) anatomical manual (illus. 12) and connections between those images and their Western counterparts.

Part Three, 'Anatomy and Artists', examines the role of professional artists in the creation, dissemination and popularization of anatomical illustrations, and the eventual collaborations between artists and anatomists that would fundamentally change image-making in Europe. Chapter Five investigates the different types of illustrations created by professional artists for anatomical texts. Initially, the increasing demand for luxury books drove workshop illuminators to devise creative and entertaining illuminations as textual dividers in medical manuscripts; eventually, professional artists became anatomists themselves, attending human dissections and engaging with medical writings to produce their images. Finally, Chapter Six focuses on the establishment and evolution of the iconography of a single image, the dissection scene, across manuscript and print in the late fifteenth and early sixteenth centuries. The arrival of Vesalius, with his richly ironic and engaging dissection scene frontispiece (see illus. 41) to *De humani corporis fabrica* (*On the Fabric of the Human Body*) of 1543, bookends one hundred years of changes in the role of printed anatomical images as epistemic tools.

Many of the diagrams presented here have not benefitted from previous study. Those that have were mostly used as evidence in specific stylistic arguments or as sidenotes in broader medical or scientific surveys, divorced from the context of other anatomical

illuminations or anatomical learning in general. This book aims
to establish medieval anatomical imagery as its own visual language, a partnership between word and graphic that was both
instructive and visually pleasing. Although the images are comparatively rare and stylistically diverse, all are united by a desire
to communicate information about the form and function of
the body's interior. Too long overlooked, they reveal much about
the ways in which medieval people considered their physical
selves and the variety of stylistic modes they used to translate
those ideas into graphic form.

PART I

ANATOMY AND COSMOS

ONE

Spiritual Anatomy
and the Monastery

In 1158 two monks of the Benedictine abbey of St George
in Prüfening, Bavaria – Swicher, a scribe, and Wolfger, a
librarian – recorded their pleasure at completing an arduous
task with satisfying rapidity: the copying of a lengthy encyclopaedic dictionary known as the *Glossarium Salomonis* (Salomon
Glossaries) onto some two hundred parchment folios, measuring
nearly 60 centimetres (2 ft) tall and 30 centimetres (1 ft) wide
(Munich, Bayerische Staatsbibliothek, Clm 13002). Accompanying the *Glossarium* were additional tools for the intellectual
enrichment of the monks of their community, including a dictionary of Greek and Latin words and short commentaries on
Old and New Testament books. The completion of this large
manuscript was an important achievement for the members of
the thriving young writing workshop (known as a scriptorium),
keen to build up its monastic library.[1] The sheer size of the
manuscript indicates that it was already considered to be a significant production by the monastery. However, even after
Swicher finished copying the texts, it was determined that the
manuscript needed something more. Eight years later, a booklet
of four bifolia of six visual vignettes was added to the front of
the book: moralizing and spiritual diagrams, including a series
of five squatting full-body figures, each revealing within its outlines the veins, arteries, bones, nerves and muscles respectively
(see illus. 2, 3).

These five diagrams, known collectively as the Five-Figure Series, are the first human anatomical images created in Europe.[2] What is more, they were significant enough to the community of monks at Prüfening to be included among the large and impressive diagrams at the start of an important collection of texts. Immediately preceding the anatomical figures are diagrams of a medical procedure called cautery, in which hot irons were applied to different parts of the body based on times of the month and year in an effort to draw out bad humours, and so

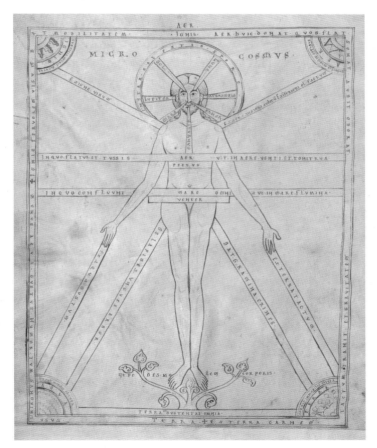

15 Microcosm, preceding *Glossarium Salomonis* (c. 1165).

they are not the only medically relevant images in the book. But the rest of the images are directly connected to the moral and spiritual life of the Prüfening community. Although the folios have since been reordered, the cycle originally began with what is considered to be the earliest diagram of the body as the microcosm (illus. 15), followed by the cautery and anatomical images, a diptych of the Vices and Virtues in three registers, and an excerpt from the English monk and author Bede (d. 735) with a drawing of Jerusalem. The series ends with an image of a scroll held aloft by angels and topped by Christ detailing the history and treasured holdings of the monastery, including its books.[3] How did the anatomical images, with no clear religious undertones or signifiers, come to be included in this particularly important product of the hands of the monks of Prüfening?

Although the Prüfening anatomical figures have no evident precedent, other types of medical and scientific diagrams flourished alongside religious texts and images in monastic manuscripts during this period, notably those depicting astronomy and the universe, maps and mathematic and computistic theories.[4] The distillation of complicated ideas into linear graphics was used for many areas of knowledge in the early Middle Ages. The Five-Figure Series is a visual translation of the anatomical theories of the foremost established medical authority of the time, Galen, which are summarized by the brief text that accompanies the images, the *Historia incisionis* (Account of Incision). Its preface begins:

> In the name of the Father, and of the Son, and of the
> Holy Spirit, here begins the account of incision described
> by Galen, most expert of physicians: vein after vein, bone
> after bone, muscle after muscle, nerve after nerve, and
> he described them as they are and separated one from the
> other, in order that the observer might not accidentally

err, but might understand in its true nature those things which he can see. Thus the first description is of the arteries; the second, the veins; the third, of the position of the bones; the fourth, the nerves; the fifth, the muscles; the sixth, the genitals; the seventh, the stomach, liver, and belly; the eighth, the womb; the ninth, the brain and the eyes.[5]

Galen posited that the body's major systems could be divided into two categories. The first five listed here – arteries, veins, bones, nerves and muscles – he considered to be the 'simples', the basic materials that make up the rest of the body. Systems six to nine are the 'compound' (also known as 'complex' or 'organic'), which the simples combined to make: the male and female reproductive systems, the stomach and internal organs, and the brain and ocular system.

The Prüfening series – featuring the five simple systems patterned on the same ideal, sterilized body – neatly communicates the positioning of each system. Each image is accompanied by its own brief description of the system's main function, and the vein and artery figures include depictions of organs important to the operation of each system. For example, the text surrounding the vein figure explains that four large veins originate in the liver, and indeed, the five-lobed liver features prominently in the abdomen. Veins emanate from there to bring blood flow to the head, other vital internal organs, and to the arms, hands, legs and feet. One of the major veins extending from the liver ascends to the diaphragm, rendered as two concentric circles in the upper chest, and from there, the description tells us, blood spreads throughout the torso. The other organs pictured are the abstracted intestinal tract, which begins with the stomach at the top and curves down to the colon, and the teardrop-shaped spleen attached to its upper right side.

Many who have considered these anatomical images believe they are copies of a now-lost late antique tradition. Most medical imagery dating from this period was inherited rather than original, as is demonstrably the case with the cautery images. However, we cannot entirely rule out the possibility that the monks of Prüfening created the Five-Figure Series themselves. The prefatory image cycle includes other drawings that appear to have been original products of the Prüfening scriptorium, including the microcosm image and the diptych of the Vices and Virtues.[6] But either as copies of an older tradition or as innovations of the Prüfening monks, determining why these anatomical images were significant to a twelfth-century monastic community requires an examination of the purpose of medical texts and images for western European monks in general and the place of medicine within the medieval monastery. The Five-Figure Series and a related, slightly later set of organ diagrams are the only anatomical images known to have emerged from monastic scriptoria. This chapter will explore these images as creations by and for monks, delving into the relationship between the body, medical learning and religion in monastic manuscripts.

Monks and Medical Knowledge

Theoretical and practical medicine were both integral aspects of monastic life. The earliest monastic communities were established in western Europe in the sixth century; Benedict of Nursia (c. 480–543 or 547) founded the first monastery at Monte Cassino in 529. His directive for monastic life, the *Rule of Saint Benedict*, dictated that a monk had to eschew all worldly goods and status and commit to living a simple and austere life of contemplation and service in an enclosed community. Monasteries were designed to be entirely self-sufficient, and labour included farming, animal husbandry and manufacture of any necessary goods, such as clothing. Monks devoted their time to worshipping Christ through prayer (through following the Liturgy of the Hours), divine reading (an active endeavour that entailed reading, meditating and praying on scripture) and manual labour. Benedict's *Rule* also stipulated that care of the sick was of paramount importance, through not only spiritual means, but practical ones as well: 'Before all things and above all things, care must be taken of the sick, so that they will be served as if they were Christ in person.'[7] Benedict instructed that the sick be allowed frequent baths and meat to eat to more quickly regain their strength, and that they should be cared for in a separate part of the monastery (the infirmary). In addition to these directives, most monastic gardens contained herbs and other plants with healing properties to be used in medicines and poultices, drawing on information contained in herbal manuscripts.

To what extent did monks and nuns provide medical attention to their brethren and beyond? It varied from place to place. In some places, care for the sick included caring for lay members of the community, as well as some laypeople not affiliated with the monastery. Although evidence suggests that monks received medical attention from laypeople outside of their communities, calling in the expertise of local physicians, surgeons, apothecaries and phlebotomists (to draw blood to keep the humours in balance), it seems that most of these roles were filled by skilled members of their own enclosures. In the later Middle Ages, monks and nuns became instrumental in the operation of hospitals for laypeople.[8]

Although many aspects of practical medicine required training through experience, certain medical procedures required book learning, especially when it came to bloodletting, which drew upon Hippocratic teachings on the balance of the four humours and an understanding of the relationships between parts of the body and the cosmos. The production and copying of texts, including medical ones, were central activities of monastic life, and monasteries were responsible for much of the circulation of medical knowledge before universities. From locating and borrowing the books to producing copies, the process of augmenting a monastic library was an arduous and serious task. The importance of actively copying texts, decorating them and making books as a spiritual exercise was enumerated by the earliest monastic writers as crucial aspects of a monk's devotional duties. As the early Roman monk Cassiodorus (*c.* 485–*c.* 585) wrote in his influential guide to the education and work of monks, *On Institutions of Divine and Secular Learning*: 'Many things indeed can be said of this outstanding art, but it is enough to say that they are called scribes who serve the balance and justice of the Lord.'[9] In the same chapter, Cassiodorus also emphasizes the importance of 'covering the loveliness of sacred letters with external beauty', that is, decorating the texts and binding them in ornate covers. Secular artists who were recognized for their abilities as illuminators were hired by monks as early as the twelfth century, and by the late Middle Ages, many monastic communities outsourced manuscript production to professional scriptoria.[10] Each text chosen for the laborious and expensive process, in-house and as external commissions, would have been identified as a useful and important addition to a monastic library.

Western medicine was forever altered by the introduction of Islamic works, mostly through the efforts of one immigrant monk: Constantine the African (d. before 1098/9).[11] Although details of his life are scarce, we know he was a merchant from northern Africa who was evidently astonished, upon arriving in Italy, to discover the locals had no treatises on urine. The art of diagnosing illness through examining the colour, smell, consistency and even taste of a patient's urine – known as urinoscopy – was a fundamental aspect of classical and Middle Eastern medicine, enough so that Constantine found the lack of Latin urinoscopy treatises to be an appalling lacuna. Despite his imperfect mastery of Latin, he joined the Benedictine order at Monte Cassino and made it his life's mission to translate as many Arabic medical writings as possible. He is known to have produced at least two dozen works and had a hand in or supervised several more. His most famous translation, the *Pantegni*, was a rendition of al-Majusi's 'Kitāb Kāmil aṣ-Ṣinā'a aṭ-Ṭibbiyya (Complete Book of the Medical Art), an encyclopaedia of medical theory mostly based on Galen's writings. Two of the *Pantegni*'s ten books were dedicated to anatomy, representing the most advanced knowledge of the subject available in the West from the end of the eleventh century until approximately the late twelfth. Constantine's translations were popular within his lifetime and had circulated as far as England only a few decades after his death.

Although the earliest anatomical images may have been created at Prüfening in Bavaria, the Galenic theories summarized by the *Historia incisionis* can almost certainly be traced back to southern Italy and Constantine's oeuvre. There is no evidence of illustration in the medical works he translated, but close inspection of the *Historia incisionis* has uncovered a link to Constantine's *De placitis Hippocratis et Platonis* (On the Concordance of Hippocrates and Plato), a treatise by Galen thought to be unknown in western Europe until the Renaissance.[12] The *De placitis* is notable as one of the most complete summaries of Galen's anatomical writings and specifically discusses the positions of the veins and arteries, and in particular the origin of the arteries in the left ventricle of the heart. The *De placitis* includes (in its original Greek) a section describing the arteries as branches of a tree, language that is directly echoed in the *Historia incisionis* but nowhere else in twelfth-century sources.[13] Constantine is recorded as having translated the *De placitis* by both of his biographers at Monte Cassino, although there are no surviving manuscript witnesses. While it is risky to venture too far into the realms of conjecture, if the *Historia incisionis* was indeed composed based on a now-lost copy of Constantine's translation of the *De placitis*, it was probably written in the Cassinese environs and eventually circulated through Benedictine monastic communities to Germany. It is not unreasonable to speculate that the treatise was either appended to existing illustrations, or was given original illustrations by Swicher and his fellow monks at Prüfening, and then circulated throughout Germany, Italy, England and beyond.

Anatomy and Art at Prüfening

Founded in 1109 by Bishop Otto 1 of Bamburg (r. 1106–39) and settled by monks from the Swabian monastery of Hirsau, Prüfening grew quickly to compete with older nearby houses. The zeal of the Prüfening monks to augment their library is well-documented by contemporary sources: in addition to serving as the librarian, Wolfger also took it upon himself to record the biographies of many of the monks of Prüfening, including when they arrived, any works they produced and if they left the community. His writings and the numerous surviving manuscripts made at Prüfening during that time indicate a vibrant community of brothers committed to building a library of important texts. They devoted extensive energy and resources to the lengthy and layered process of bookmaking. They also clearly had an interest in Galenic medical theories and the regulation of the humours through cautery, a procedure that often went hand-in-hand with the popular process of bloodletting.

Why did the Prüfening monks choose these particular images in this particular order in combination with this particular text? In the Prüfening manuscript, the anatomical (and cautery) images form part of a 'spiritual encyclopaedia', to borrow Fritz

Saxl's term, of scientific material alongside religious.[14] Although contemporary viewers might consider the Five-Figure Series and anatomical treatise 'secular' in comparison with the explicitly religious images and texts in the manuscript, the Prüfening monks would have viewed them as vehicles to encourage divine contemplation, and the act of copying them a vital piece of their monastic duties. The monks had access to what they believed were Galen's writings on the processes of the body's interior, and as a respected authority, Galen's theories were acceptable as a means for greater understanding of their world. There was no perceived difference between religion and science, especially not as we conceive of those two terms today. Indeed, the concept of 'science' in the modern sense – as a field that is provable by experimentation – did not exist. Rather, a *scientia* was someone's knowledge of a particular subject, like natural philosophy, often drawn from recognized authorities and adapted to contemporary emphasis on pious contemplation. Inspiring deliberation of the physical body and the spiritual, the anatomical images and text also potentially represent a specific meditative process devised to encourage divine stimulation for the brothers.[15] In fact, we can see the importance of the individual in the careful recording of names of the Prüfening monks involved in the manuscript's production. If a Prüfening monk was inspired to create his own meditation (*meditatio*) image cycle, he had not only the freedom to do so, but the confidence that God and his brethren would appreciate his efforts.

Monks as Anatomical Creators Beyond Prüfening

The *Historia incisionis* and Five-Figure Series did not sit undisturbed in Prüfening's library collecting dust. The monastery was proud of the manuscript its scribes had laboriously copied, so much so that they loaned it to the nearby monastery of Scheyern in the early thirteenth century, where it was reproduced almost in its entirety and on a similar scale (Munich, Bayerische Staatsbibliothek, Clm 17403).[16] The Scheyern monks added other medical materials, including a herbal and list of medical terms, to their copy of the Prüfening contents. The Five-Figure Series thus entered into the monastic practice of sharing and copying to disseminate knowledge and was reproduced in all or in part across Europe over the next three centuries.[17]

Approximately forty years after the Prüfening manuscript was made, the Five-Figure Series and *Historia incisionis* appeared in England, but this time with the addition of four abstracted diagrams representing Galen's compound organ systems as well. All nine drawings occupy their own page in a small booklet of four bifolia that was later added to a mid-fifteenth-century compilation of miscellaneous medical texts from the Premonstratensian abbey of Hagnaby in Lincolnshire (Cambridge, Gonville and Caius College, MS 190/223).[18] Since it ended up in a monastic setting, it is probable – especially given the Benedictine origins of the Prüfening manuscript – that the Cambridge booklet was initially created in a monastic, likely Benedictine scriptorium. The small and portable nature of the booklet, as well as the damage to the exterior folios, suggests that it circulated independently before settling at Hagnaby. In any case, the monks at Hagnaby placed the anatomical booklet before copies of medical texts that were popular in mid-fifteenth-century England, including a good amount of surgical material. Here we see the alliance between anatomy and surgery, two subjects that became inextricably linked in university medical curricula between the time of the Cambridge booklet's creation and its absorption into this particular manuscript.

The booklet begins with the Five-Figure Series (two of which can be seen in illustrations 16 and 17), progressing in the same order found in the Prüfening version and with an almost identical distribution of the *Historia incisionis* text surrounding the figures. These five are followed by diagrams of the male genitalia (the sixth system; see illus. 4), the stomach and internal organs (the seventh system; illus. 5), the female reproductive system (eighth; illus. 18) and the brain and ocular system (ninth; illus. 19).[19] Given that the Galenic text mentions nine systems, these images and the *Historia incisionis* have been collectively called the Nine-Figure Series. The Nine-Figure Series only appears as a whole in two other manuscripts, and there is just one instance of the four compound organ diagrams travelling without their more popular Five-Figure brethren.[20] How these four images – so different stylistically to the Five-Figure Series – came to be combined with the *Historia incisionis* text and five simple systems is unknown. The brain and ocular image is similar to a roughly contemporary Middle Eastern diagram (see illus. 8), which indicates a common Islamic or late antique ancestor, but the Islamic version only features the ocular and nasal system, while the Cambridge diagram includes a colourful depiction of the brain as well.

Although they are the only anatomical images to take this form, these renderings of the four compound organs, distilled into geometric, abstract shapes, reflect a larger tradition of schematic scientific diagrams created in the early Middle Ages.[21] The artist(s) turned to abstraction to communicate complicated workings and structures in simplified, memorable forms. The Five-Figure Series – patterned on a template of the human body – is easily relatable to the viewer, but the abstracted organ forms forgo the confines of the body to convey not only their physical attributes but their physiological processes as well, through a combination of oversimplification and impossible perspectives.[22] These images were not meant to tell the reader exactly where each organ is situated within the body; they employ inorganic shapes to express why a particular system was important, rather than where it was located. Eschewing anatomical reality in

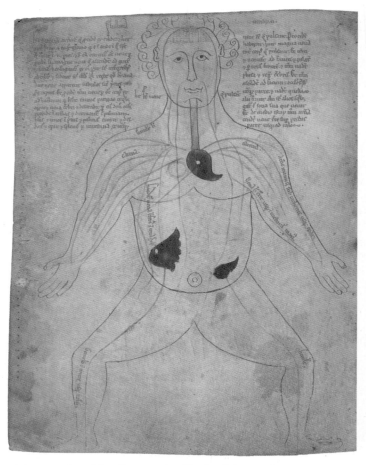

16 Arteries, from *Miscellanea medica* [England] (c. 1200).

favour of abstract forms allowed the artist(s) to express ideas over physical truths, freeing them to make graphic decisions that bent the bounds of nature. In keeping with most scientific diagrams of the high Middle Ages, communication of a concept was prioritized over representation of nature.

The Cambridge scribe added a small legend within the text between the legs of the bone figure (illus. 17), set between crosses, reading 'The picture says the rest' (*reliquam dicit pictura*). This

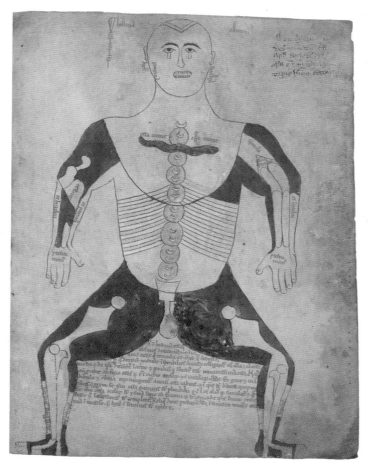

17 Bones, from *Miscellanea medica* [England] (*c.* 1200).

brief phrase represents a concrete indication of the perceived importance of the images by the scribe, as well as the inverse: the texts were crucial in understanding the complicated structures of the body's interior.[23] The placements of captions and descriptions within and around the forms further elucidate their function. Rather than requiring longer prose explanations, like those accompanying the figurative Five-Figure Series, word and shape work together to communicate physiology for the four

compound systems. The required physical interaction needed
to access these particular unions between word and image is striking; the placement of the descriptions forces the reader to either
shift his or her body, or to turn the image (and thus the codex)
to read words inserted sideways and upside-down. The image
both describes movement and requires movement on the reader's behalf to fully engage with it. This action is most notably
required by the first complex system, a bisected view of the male
reproductive system (see illus. 4).[24] The image is large, organized
and colourful, filling the entire folio. The penis and testes are
framed by a double border, the outer of which is decorated with
alternating solid paint or stripes. The inner border is mostly filled
with text, and along with the captions woven within the drawing,
the words describe the function of the penis and the movement
of the semen, which, it explains, descends from the spine and
gathers in the testes.

Contemporary scholars have argued this image would have
been easily recognizable to its male audience; it is clear and relatable to their own bodies, especially when compared to the obscure
shapes that make up the female reproductive system (illus. 18).[25]
The female system is likewise organized and symmetrical, but far
less description accompanies it than the male, and it is not immediately identifiable. Both would have been important much
literature was devoted to the roles of the male and female in
reproduction. The medieval conception of the female reproductive system usually posited that the uterus was seven-celled: three
cells on the right were chambers for male foetuses, three cells on
the left were for females and one in the centre was for an intersex
foetus. However, in the Nine-Figure Series diagram, the uterus is
bicornate ('two-horned'), a term that stems from Aristotelian
language.[26] The drawing is accented by rose-and-white pig-
ments, and the overall impression is one of symmetry, elegance
and an effort at geometrical precision. The captions describe the

movement of the female seed, explaining it comes from the ovaries
(called *testiculi*, and understood to function as the female equivalent of male testicles), along with the positions of the muscles,
flow of blood and other physiological aspects of the system. The
Nine-Figure Series image is the only version of the female reproductive system to feature the bicornate uterus as opposed to the
seven-celled.

The final abstract diagram, the brain and ocular system, veers
even more deeply into abstraction and has very little in the way
of textual labels (illus. 19). The medieval understanding of the
brain drew upon a long history of discussing its capabilities and
position within the hierarchy of the body.[27] By the early Middle
Ages, the brain was considered to be encased by a hard layer
(*dura mater*) and a soft layer (*pia mater*) and to have three principal sections, known as cells, which were responsible for the
three mental faculties. The anterior ventricle was the site of the
imagination, reason resided in the middle and memory lay in
the posterior. The Cambridge diagram only includes a representation of one of the three cells (reason) and no real elaboration
or explanation of the function of the parts of the brain, assuming
either an informed audience or a lack of further textual support
from available sources. The colourful shapes of the brain are
drawn above what is potentially a representation of the forehead,
and the two ocular nerves descend from there to the eyeballs,
cutting through four multicoloured tunics of the eye. The nasal
passageway ends in a stylized outline drawing of the nose.[28]
This type of brain diagram is rare; while diagrams of the *mind*
were relatively common (usually pictured within a living head
and upper torso) alongside philosophical texts, diagrams of the
anatomy of the brain were unusual.[29]

More fragmented and less abstracted is the seventh system,
the stomach and internal viscera (see illus. 5).[30] Instead of presenting a view of an abdomen, each organ situated inside in its

respective position, the readers are shown what might be a dissector's table scattered with viscera. There are alternative views, some exterior and some interior of the same organs. The artist has drawn a simplified, schematic four-chambered stomach at top left, complete with a brief description describing the stomach's role as an 'oven' in which food is cooked and then discarded to the digestive tract. The rest of the folio displays ten other

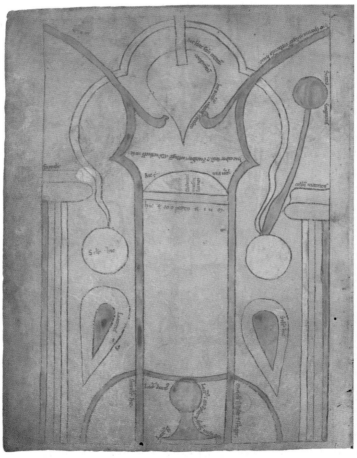

18, 19 Female reproductive system (above), and brain and ocular system (opposite), from *Miscellanea medica* [England] (*c.* 1200).

organs of the chest and abdomen, from the recognizable half-moon pair of kidneys on the right edge to the entirely abstracted trachea fitting into the lungs directly above. There are two views of the brown, five-lobed liver and gallbladder, one of which shows the liver's position wrapped around the stomach; a bright red heart with two lobes protruding like ears; and an uncoloured sketch of the gallbladder on its own. Many of these renderings

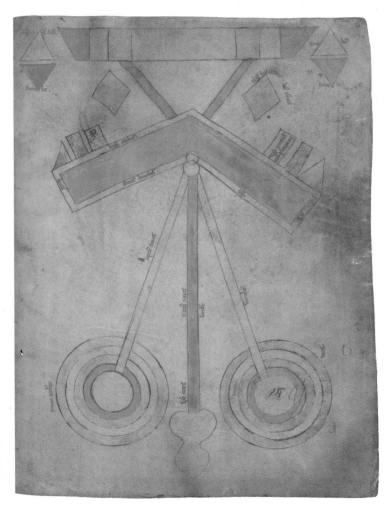

are impossible to decipher without the help of the captions. The combination of these figures on a single folio, ranging from the completely abstract to the slightly more mimetic, indicates a desire on the part of the artist to present the reader with as many tools for understanding the parts as possible. Given the absence of a prose text devoted to describing the organs of the abdomen, it seems likely the artist hoped multiple perspectives could further elucidate their shapes and functions.

Unlike the Prüfening scriptorium, the fifteenth-century Hagnaby monks did not combine the Cambridge anatomical booklet with religious materials, but rather they – already in possession of a group of surgical texts – chose to keep anatomy and surgery together as reference materials. While the position of the images in the Prüfening manuscript indicates they facilitated some religious contemplation, the Cambridge Nine-Figure Series could have served a more straightforwardly medical role, able to be carried around freely and consulted easily. One could visualize the interior while consulting the descriptions of the surgical procedures outlined in the pages following.

Monks and University Anatomy

At the time of the Prüfening manuscript's production in the second half of the twelfth century, the first universities were barely more than loose communities of students, many of them clerics, designed in the image of monasteries.[31] The earliest medical faculties were incorporated into universities in the late thirteenth century, and while most professional doctors and surgeons were laypeople, clerics were allowed to both study and teach scholastic medicine. Although Salerno was renowned as a centre of medical learning between the late eleventh and early thirteenth centuries, it waned in influence in the beginning of the thirteenth century and no formal university was established

in the city until the second half of the century. But it was at
Salerno that Constantine's works, produced at nearby Monte
Cassino, and others were compiled into the fundamental text-
book of university medical learning, known collectively as the
Articella (Little Art). The *Articella* was comprised of seven short
texts by medical authorities largely based around the *Isagoge*
(Introduction), Constantine's translation of the *Masâ'il fi-tibb*
(Questions on Medicine) by Hunayn ibn Ishâq (809–887),
which was itself a summary of Galen's *Art of Medicine* (also known
in the Latin West as the *Tegni*, from the Greek *techne*, meaning
'art').[32] The *Articella* was combined with several Hippocratic
diagnostic texts and two Byzantine treatises on urine and the
pulses to make up a largely practical, easily understood compilation that formed the backbone of medieval medical learning.[33]

The universities of Bologna, Paris and Montpellier became
the most famous places to study medicine. There were also
medical faculties at Oxford and Cambridge, but the subject was
not nearly as popular, and there are few records of masters –
teachers who attracted students on an individual basis due to
their reputations as experts in certain subjects – at either university until the late fourteenth century.[34] The Church, as the
ultimate authority over universities, played a large role in the
formation of medicine as a professional discipline: in Paris by
the mid-fourteenth century, all medical licences were awarded
by the chancellor, the archbishop of Paris's secretary and traditional master of the schools, following a student's successful
study of a recognized medical curriculum. The Church ensured
the legitimacy of the masters by granting them licence to practice and teach medicine. Many of the masters at the University
of Paris were members of the clergy, and the same appears to be
true for Oxford and Cambridge. Furthermore, the movement
of masters and students between the three universities in the
thirteenth century is well documented. It is also why we see the

circulation of medical texts between the three so often; when a master decided to leave his university in favour of another, he usually took with him both his students and his books.

As universities expanded, so too did the volume of manuscripts copied, as the knowledge possessed by monks moved outside of their communities. In addition to their circulation through Benedictine monastic houses, the *Historia incisionis* and Nine-Figure Series likely travelled in university settings, in a portable booklet like the Cambridge manuscript, or with popular medical texts as mnemonic tools, helpful to students in memorizing complicated descriptions of physiology.[35] Following the creation of the Nine-Figure Series in the Cambridge manuscript in England around 1200, the four organ diagrams appear without the Five-Figure Series in a two-bifolia parchment booklet, folded together rather than bound, one bifolium of which is in Pisa (Biblioteca Universitaria, MS 735).[36] The other is in a private collection in Switzerland, dated to the second quarter of the thirteenth century, probably of Italian origin.[37] Nothing is securely known about the production of the booklet, but the sketched cautery and anatomical diagrams and unbound parchment leaves, once folded into quarters, indicate it was used as a compact, handy reference guide for a medical student or teacher.

The same nine images and text appear in more decorative form at the end of the thirteenth century in England (Oxford, Bodleian Library, MS Ashmole 399) alongside an array of medical texts and images (illus. 20–22, 37).[38] Ashmole 399 includes extensive writings on gynaecology, obstetrics and reproduction, as well as other popular texts, including a treatise on the pulses and miscellaneous recipes. Although there is no sure indication of its provenance, it seems likely it was made for a clerical patron due to the inclusion of tools for computing Easter dates as well as depictions of both a lay physician and a tonsured helper in a miniature cycle.

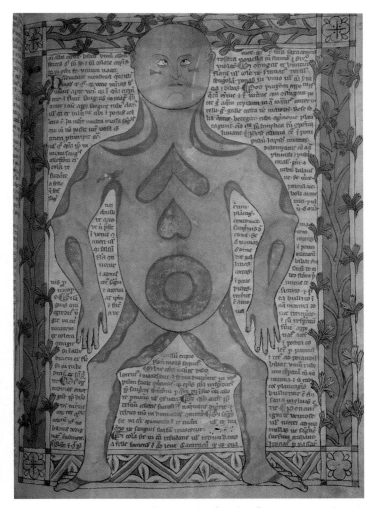

20 Muscle figure, from *Miscellanea medica* [England] (c. 1250–1310).

The Nine-Figure Series in Ashmole 399 is similar enough to the images in the Cambridge booklet that it is likely they were a direct copy. As in the Cambridge version, each of the Ashmole Five-Figure Series is allotted a full folio, surrounded by colourful foliate borders (illus. 20). Originally, they were uncrowded by text; the writing that now occupies the space around them is unrelated. The *Historia incisionis* descriptions were copied onto the verso of the preceding folio – so that, when opened, both were laid out in front of the reader – and begun with a large gold initial. The Ashmole 'men' are especially unique, delightfully cartoonish in a way that evokes a ludic playfulness. In addition to their crossed eyes, the five squatting figures are all tinted with a grey wash that is slightly darker than the parchment, vaguely corpse-like. Their large heads, hands and delicately arched feet extend over the vibrant leafy borders, which provide a clue to the approximate time of production; similar designs can be found in contemporary stained glass, common between the period of circa 1270–1320.[39] While less ornate, the four compound systems are also given plenty of space, enlarged and sometimes rendered with more of an effort at naturalism than those on the Cambridge organ leaf (especially the heart; illus. 21). The Ashmole maker(s) chose not to clutter the drawings even with the brief labels that accompany their Cambridge predecessors, save for alongside the female reproductive system (illus. 22), which does not appear with the other abstracted organs diagrams, but instead was inserted among the other gynaecological and obstetrical materials at the start of the manuscript. Ashmole 399 also famously includes a unique miniature cycle depicting the disease, treatment, death and graphic autopsy of a woman, treated by a physician who is assisted by a tonsured cleric (see illus. 37). The cycle will be discussed in more detail presently, but for now, the presence of the monk indicates both the relationship between monks and lay medical practitioners in the mid-thirteenth century, working together to provide treatment, as well as the potential audience of the manuscript itself.[40]

When the Nine-Figure Series last appears (London, Wellcome Library, MS 49; illus. 23–4, 30, 63), the decorative and the sacred are again united in a book made for a monkish audience. Dated to approximately 1425, the codex is notable for several reasons,

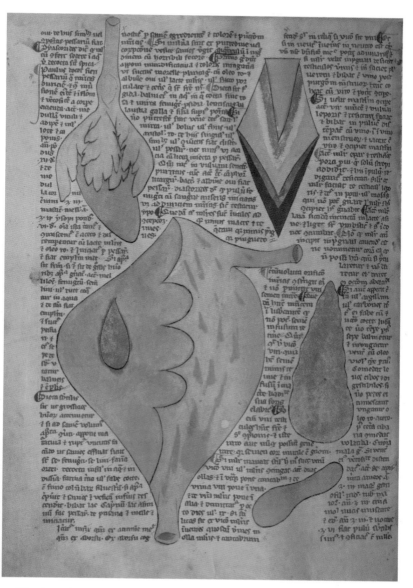

21 The heart (upper left), trachaea? (upper right), stomach covered by
five-lobed liver and gallbladder (center), gallbladder (middle right) and
spleen (bottom right), from *Miscellanea medica* [England] (c. 1250–1310).

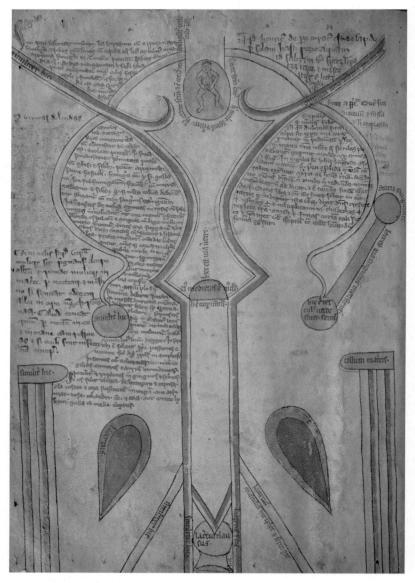

22 Female reproductive system, from *Miscellanea medica* [England] (*c.* 1250–1310).

foremost among them the inclusion of a section on medicine and anatomy in the middle of a large, expensive religious and moralizing compendium that includes treatises for monks detailing how to live a good spiritual life.[41] Nothing concrete is known about the volume's provenance before the eighteenth century, but it was most likely produced in Germany given the presence of German texts. The manuscript's considerable size and organization, with each block of text arranged thoughtfully around the delicately uniform tinted images, indicates a professional scriptorium produced the manuscript for a clerical audience.

The Wellcome Five-Figure Series has been updated to more naturalistic poses, casually standing on grassy knolls (illus. 23–4), and the entire Nine-Figure Series is supplemented by newer, full-body imagery presenting a more cohesive view of the medical body. While the abstract diagrams are still difficult to understand without textual aid, the creative forces behind their inclusion in the Wellcome volume took steps to demystify them. First, the codex's planners entirely omitted the most inscrutable, the diagram of the brain and ocular system. They also streamlined the amount of standalone abdomen organ diagrams, only including a single image of those that had featured multiple views and situating them next to the vein man of the Five-Figures, which includes several of the organs pictured within the context of the body (illus. 63). The artists also chose to unite all reproductive materials on the same folio, so that the womb is accompanied by the male diagram and representations of the foetal positions in the womb (illus. 24), and further elucidated by the presence of a large Disease Woman diagram on the facing page (see illus. 30), who demonstrates the various parts within her torso.

While the anatomical material in the Wellcome manuscript is unique for the time – it post-dates the second oldest manuscript to include all of the Nine-Figure Series by nearly two centuries – if we consider the volume in light of the earlier

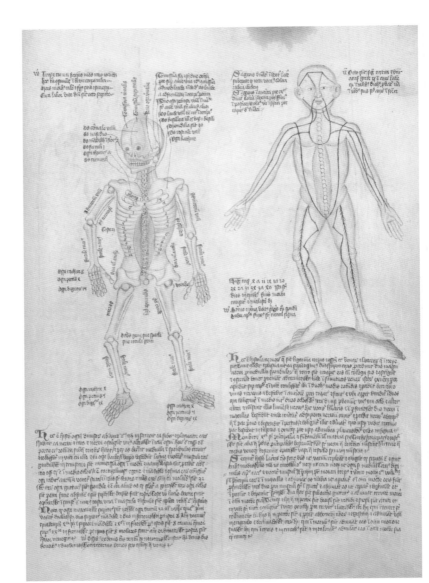

23 Bone figure (left) and nerve figure (right), from the 'Wellcome Apocalypse' (c. 1425).

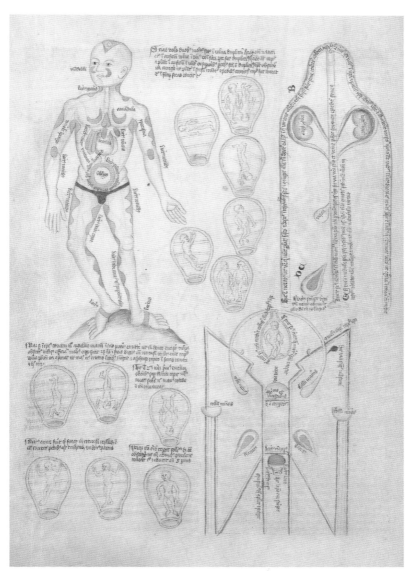

24 Muscle figure, foetus-in-utero diagrams and male and female
reproductive systems, from the 'Wellcome Apocalypse' (*c.* 1425).

examples of these anatomical images, there is in fact nothing strange about it.[42] The three earlier examples were also most likely made in monastic contexts, and although the amount of gynaecological material in the Wellcome version is pronounced, it would not have been considered an unusual addition to a cleric or clerical institution's library. Indeed, we can see echoes of this acceptance of the medical with the spiritual in the Prüfening and Scheyern codices; along with the Wellcome, all three incorporate medical and religious imagery, specifically the Virtues and Vices, and demonstrate – across three hundred years – the breadth of medical learning in monasteries, of which anatomy formed a part. In Wellcome MS 49, we can again see the easy symbiotic relationship between science and Christianity, art and medicine.

* * *

Monasteries were the cradles of European anatomy: the first anatomical images, known as the Five-Figure Series, were drawn by monks in Bavaria in 1165, and it was a monk of Monte Cassino, Constantine the African, who translated the anatomical texts that would come to dominate the literature of the Middle Ages. Learning anatomy was not a significant aspect of monastic medicine, but the texts and images monks copied and created served an important purpose in their intellectual and spiritual lives, encouraging meditation on the relationship between the physical body and the cosmic, the micro and the macro. The sexless, perfected body template used for the Five-Figure Series allowed a monk to consider his own interior, and the abstracted organ diagrams of the four compound figures that accompanied the Five-Figure Series likewise compartmentalized complicated physiological theories into orderly geometries. As will be explored in the next chapter, understanding the connection between the body and the universe became increasingly important in medical practice during the high and later Middle Ages. The appearance of the earliest anatomical bodies alongside the earliest microcosm image by the Prüfening monks marks the visual start of the interaction between anatomy and cosmology in medieval medicine.

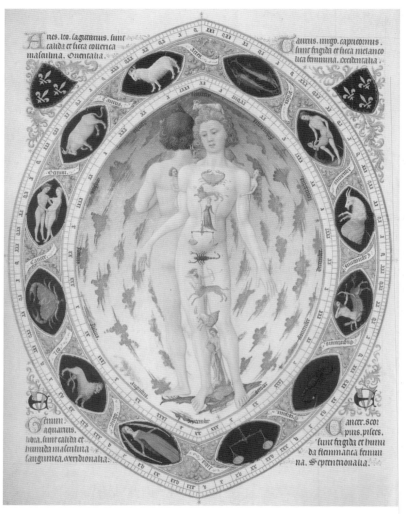

25 Zodiac figure, from the *Très riches heures* of the Duke of Berry (c. 1413).

TWO

Blood and Stars:
Anatomical Astrology

The union of spiritual and anatomical material in the Prüfening manuscript indicates the importance of the relationship between the body and the cosmos in medieval medical practice. Beyond the significance of prayer and faith as spiritual treatments for disease and illness, there was an ancient, pre-Christian philosophical undercurrent running through learned medieval medicine that linked the physical body to forces at work in the wider universe.[1] Classical Greek thinkers introduced the concepts of microcosm and macrocosm, or 'little universe' and 'big universe', by arguing that the same elemental materials make up both human beings and the wider cosmos, and so the health of the 'little universe' of the human body was subject to the movements of the larger. Effecting forces included the four elements (earth, fire, wind and water), the four qualities (hot, dry, moist and cold) , which were present in all living things, and the four seasons (spring, summer, autumn and winter), as well as the movements of the stars and planets (astrology and astronomy). This micro-macrocosm theory existed alongside the Hippocratic system of medical treatment, based on keeping the body's four humours (blood, yellow bile, black bile and phlegm) in balance through evacuation of those that became too predominant or corrupted. Later Galenic medicine taught that the management of variable external factors known as the non-naturals (food and drink, air, exercise, sleep, excretion, emotions and so on) was equally important to maintaining health and treating illness. All of these components had to be taken into consideration for effective medical treatment.

In the Middle Ages, these concepts were adapted to fit the Christian worldview, as visualized in the Prüfening image cycle.[2] The diagram of the microcosm (see illus. 15) presents the correlations between the body, the elements (drawn in the four corners of the frame), planets and humours, and derives from the combination of these ancient concepts and the biblical teaching that God created man in his own image. The diagram is balanced and harmonious, similar to Leonardo da Vinci's later Vitruvian Man in proportionality and composition, presenting the different components of the universe and their connections to the body. The body of man is at the centre of the image, nude, and although he does not have any visible internal anatomy, several of his parts are aligned with different properties: for instance, the torso cavity (*venter*) appears with the inscription *mare* or ocean, just as the chest (*pectus*) is paired with air (*aer*) and the feet with earth (*terra*). The head is aligned with the planets and fire (*ignis*). Christian theology used the body as a map, in which Christ was the head, and the body represented earthly people trying to reach Christ; the ascension of the soul to heaven was a microcosmic version of the macrocosmic event of Christ ascending to heaven.[3] Several southern German monasteries like Prüfening specialized in creating these types of spiritual diagrams, which were devised to help the viewer remember the information they presented;[4] indeed, this is the earliest to present the body as a microcosm, probably an original product of the Prüfening scriptorium.

The connection between the microcosm image and the anatomical Five-Figure Series would be furthered in diagrams that explicitly depicted the link between the interior body and the exterior forces of the universe. Through a combination of word and image, they served as memory aids and practical guides for medical students and practitioners, instructing them on how to take these links into account when providing medical care, while at the same time they were entertaining to look at and accessible for an educated and elite but not specifically medical audience. This chapter will explore those diagrams meant to aid a practitioner in controlling cosmological factors to maintain a patient's health. These fall into three main categories, all of which are seldom seen before the fourteenth century: melothesia diagrams, or those that depict the connection between astrology and the parts of the body; bloodletting figures, which demonstrate locations of veins that should be evacuated, and how to compute the best times to perform those evacuations according to the movements of the planets and stars; and images of the various afflictions of the body, their causes and how they should be treated. While there are versions of each of these images that do not include depictions of interior anatomy, we will focus on those that unambiguously show the connection between astrology, astronomy and anatomy, and how such images were understood and used by practitioners, laymen and medical students.

Melothesia Diagrams and Anatomy

The twelfth-century Prüfening diagram of the microcosm was composed before new translations from Arabic into Latin of Greek astronomical and astrological treatises, especially those by Ptolemy, in the thirteenth century turned the art of predicting effective medical remedies through astrological knowledge into a physician's most valued service.[5] As we rely today on doctors who prescribe treatments based on scientific data, the reading of a person's horoscope and subsequent treatment plan based on astrological and astronomical calculations was considered to be an exact and critical skill in the Middle Ages. The most common course of action to both treat and prevent illnesses was by regulating the humours through phlebotomy, or bloodletting. Blood was a humour itself (*sanguinis*) and was also believed to carry the other three, so evacuating blood from certain veins allowed a doctor to regulate all four humours. Cautery was another means to balance humours through applying hot irons to different points of the body, which would then scab over and ooze out ill humours (as depicted in the scenes above the Five-Figure Series diagrams in illustration 2). Like cautery, bloodletting allowed the practitioner to purge the body of bad humours and restore the patient to health with careful calculation of external factors affecting the delicate microcosm of the body. Each required the physician to know which body parts were associated with certain astronomical objects, elements and the zodiac.

Each body part was directly linked to one of the twelve zodiac signs, and each organ likewise to the planets. It was thought that blood pooled in a specific body part when the Moon moved into that part's zodiac sign, making bleeding or surgery upon it dangerous and potentially fatal. Physicians had to have a firm understanding of how to compute celestial movements to treat their patients, and many physicians' handbooks included tables and charts to help them in this endeavour.[6] Although these tools had circulated for centuries, figurative diagrams did not become popular until the late fourteenth and fifteenth centuries, when nude male bodies depicting bloodletting points and the signs of the zodiac became increasingly common. A brief text providing tips for bloodletting accompanied these images in most cases.[7] While the earliest bloodletting figures were humble – often simple line drawings appearing in collections of medical treatises (illus. 26) – zodiac figures were visually striking from the start: full-bodied men with star signs superimposed over body parts, beginning with the head (corresponding to Aries) and ending with the feet (Pisces).[8]

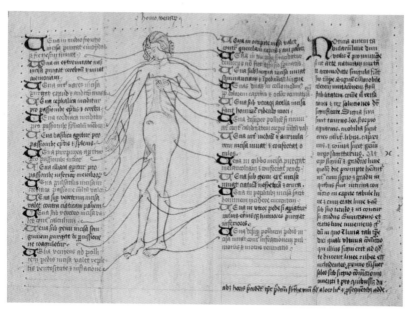

26 Bloodletting figure in an English folding almanac (mid-15th century).

Bloodletting and especially zodiac figures were not limited to medical contexts, appearing in books of hours and other religious manuscripts as well, illustrating how seamlessly astrology and astronomy fit with the Christian worldview. Perhaps the most famous example of the zodiac figure was created by a team of professional illuminators, the Limbourg Brothers, for the highly illuminated book of hours known as the *Très riches heures* of the Duke of Berry (c. 1412–16, Chantilly, Bibliothèque du musée Condé, MS 65; illus. 25). This striking diagram features a male figure in gentle contrapposto against a blue sky, clouds swirling around him like a vortex, his body covered by zodiac signs. The surrounding mandorla displays the months of the year next to additional representations of each zodiac symbol on a dark blue background. The four corners of the page describe, in Latin – above the duke's coat of arms – the ways in which the signs are grouped by their complexional (hot, cold, wet and dry), temperamental (choleric, melancholic, sanguine and phlegmatic) and cardinal properties. For example, the top left inscription tells us that 'Aries, Leo and Sagittarius are hot and dry, choleric, masculine, eastern,' and in the top right corner, almost the opposite: 'Taurus, Virgo and Capricorn are cold and dry, melancholic, female, western.'[9] This recalls the arrangements of text and image in the Prüfening microcosm diagram.

Although few were produced at the same level as the Limbourg Brothers' version, most zodiac figures also did not include representations of the internal organs, relying instead on the

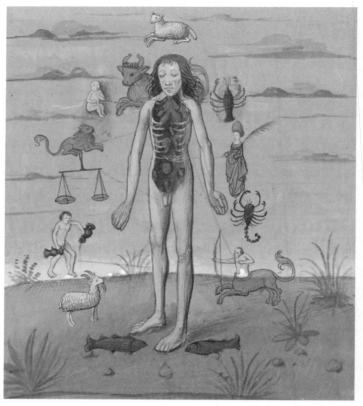

27 Zodiac anatomical figure, from Bartholomew the Englishman, *Livre des propriétés des choses* (c. 1470).

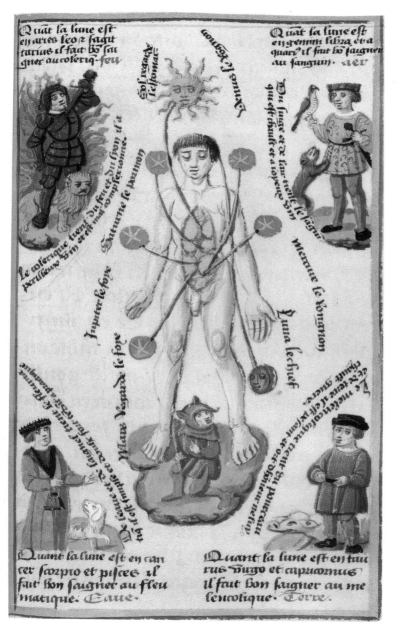

28 Planetary man, from *Le calendrier des bergers* (c. 1486).

surrounding text to explain to the reader which zodiac sign corresponded to what organ. A rare exception to this is found in a manuscript made in Bruges in approximately 1470, featuring a male figure standing in a verdant outdoor setting, his internal organs exposed, the signs of the zodiac floating in the air around him (Paris, Bibliothèque nationale de France, MS fr. 134; illus. 27). A similar image in a late fifteenth-century manuscript made in Germany that also shows the zodiac symbols framing a nude male body, making room for his chest to be opened to reveal his viscera, is from a 1488 copy of Heymandus de Veteri Busco's *Ars computistica* (Art of Computation) (London, Wellcome Library, MS 349; see illus. 1). Ropelike lines extend from each symbol to the relevant body part, showing the viewer clearly that Cancer corresponded to the stomach, Leo to the heart, Virgo to the intestines, Libra the kidneys and Scorpio the genitals. The late fifteenth-century trope of lines extending to various points on an opened body can also be seen in a slightly different type of cosmos figure, known as the planetary man. While more common in early printed books than in manuscripts, there is at least one manuscript version in a late fifteenth-century French book (Cambridge, Fitzwilliam Museum, MS 167; illus. 28). The detailed captions and images surrounding the nude figure, whose chest gapes open to display a crowded array of mostly nondescript fleshy orbs, demonstrate the planets' connection to the internal organs and when to perform bloodletting based on the position of the Moon within the zodiac signs. The men in the four corners are personifications of the four temperaments; for instance, at top left, a knight is surrounded by fire (*feu*) with a lion, and the caption below explains the properties of a choleric person.

Bloodletting Diagrams and Anatomy

Like zodiac figures, bloodletting (or phlebotomy) figures did not
often include images of the internal organs, for obvious reasons:
the practice involved a physician making a small incision into
a specific surface vein – not disturbing the organs – at certain
times of the month or year depending on the positions of the
planets and zodiac.[10] But bloodletting points were associated with
organs and a practitioner needed to know internal anatomy to
successfully deploy the therapeutic treatment. Bloodletting and
zodiac figures often travelled together; for easy consultation by
a physician, they were sometimes included in portable folded
booklets known as almanacs or calendars. Carried by physicians
and churchmen, these folded almanacs often hung from the belt,
to be consulted by the wearer like a map.[11] A fifteenth-century
English example (Wellcome MS 40; see illus. 26) shows a bloodletting figure surrounded by descriptions of when to take blood
from specific veins. The figure is pictured above a lunar table so
the user could calculate astrological movements and thus the
proper time to manage a patient's humours through phlebotomy.[12]

Although internal anatomy pictured within a bloodletting
figure was uncommon, there is one (and only one, to my knowledge) unique overlap between the bloodletting tradition and the
oldest anatomical imagery in Europe, the Five-Figure Series: a
squatting anatomical figure surrounded by a phlebotomy text
(illus. 29).[13] The image appears on a flyleaf (an older piece of used
and/or damaged parchment inserted to protect a new work) of a
copy of a popular late medieval handbook of health regimens
known as *Tacuinum sanitatis* (Maintenance of Health). *Tacuinum
sanitatis* included recommendations on how to regulate diet,
exercise and the humours for optimal well-being, based on an
eleventh-century Arabic treatise.[14] The bloodletting figure on
the flyleaf squats in the characteristic Five-Figure Series manner,

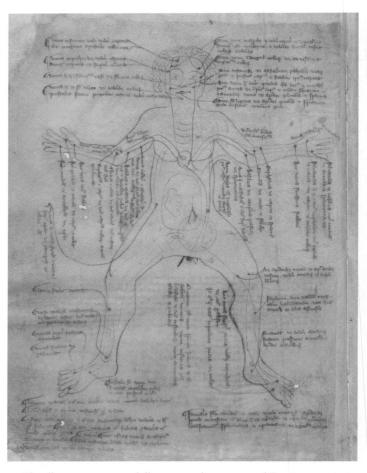

29 Bloodletting anatomical figure preceding a copy of *Tacuinum sanitatis* (c. 1400?).

and within its torso are roughly sketched outlines of the heart (in the centre of the chest) above the four-lobed liver with the gallbladder and the spleen. These three organs are the hallmarks of the artery Five-Figure Series image; however, the artist has added more bright red veins criss-crossing the body, with dark points marking the places where blood ought to be drawn. These are linked to brief descriptions of when to bleed these specific veins. Although the exact dating of this figure is unknown, the similarities are a unique testament to the adaption of the Five-Figure Series template to serve the more practical purposes associated with bloodletting imagery.

Three-Figure Series

The use of the full-body template for zodiac and bloodletting images provided a physician with a visual road map for determining treatment. But the final types of full-body figures discussed here served more as theoretical reference guides, depicting the problems that *could* befall areas of the body and how best to treat them. These were the Disease Man, the Wound Man and the Disease Woman (illus. 30), which modern historians have designated the Three-Figure Series, although they appear more often apart than they do together.[15] The Disease Man demonstrates ailments most common to men – many of which match the Disease Woman's ills – and the compellingly dramatic Wound Man image, like the one found in Wellcome MS 49 (illus. 31), showcases the many ways in which the male body could be injured through trauma or accidents. These three were popular during the fifteenth century and would make the jump to print at the turn of the sixteenth; however, the female figure was the only one shown with detailed anatomical features, while the Wound Man and Disease Man relied more heavily on external ornamentation like pustules and buboes, an axe to the upper arm or a sword through the calf. The Wound Man usually included an image of the heart, pierced by a dagger, as well as some light torso anatomy like the ribs and intestines. As is the case with the other types of images mentioned here, these figures unite word and image within the same diagram. In the case of the Three-Figure Series, their associated blocks of description provide tips for treatment of each illness or injury.

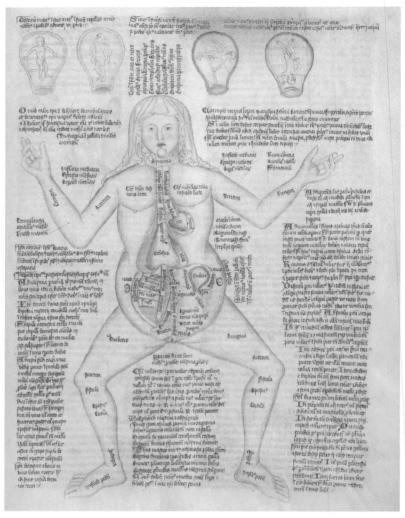

30 Disease Woman, from the 'Wellcome Apocalypse' (c. 1425).

The history of full-figured female diagrams is brief in comparison with the paradigmatic male bodies beginning with the Five-Figure Series. There are copious amounts of medical writings throughout antiquity and the Middle Ages devoted to reproduction, and the female body was valued mostly for the role

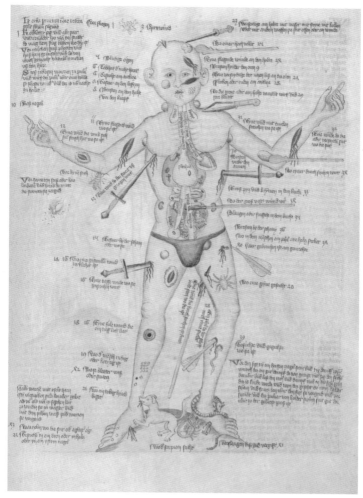

31 Wound Man, from the 'Wellcome Apocalypse' (c. 1425).

it played in the process. Thus early diagrams of female anatomy
were restricted to the positions of foetuses in the womb (see
illus. 9) and depictions of the reproductive system alone (as in
the Nine-Figure Series tradition; see illus. 18). In medieval
Europe, there are only a few other examples of full-bodied female
anatomical figures outside of the Disease Woman tradition,

drawn alongside other anatomical figures and dating to the fourteenth century.[16] However, these are one-offs. The earliest of these (see illus. 14), made around 1300 in southern France, has no captions or related text, merely presenting a modest female demonstrating her seven-celled womb.[17] Another (illus. 32) appears in a cycle of eighteen images illustrating an anatomical manual composed in mid-fourteenth-century France that we will discuss presently, and this figure has even less anatomy than the first: the seven-celled womb is the only interior organ pictured.[18]

The Disease Woman (see illus. 30) is positively packed with information in comparison to these earlier figures.[19] Included in the anatomical section of the German manuscript of circa 1425 – Wellcome MS 49 (see illus. 23–4, 30), explored in Chapter One – facing the folio with the Nine-Figure Series diagrams of the female and male reproductive systems and the foetal positions, the woman is shown with both figure and text crammed in her abdomen. The surrounding words describe how certain ailments should be treated, including bloodletting points. While most of the examples of the Disease Woman are depicted with a foetus in the womb, the Wellcome woman merely has the word 'embrio' as a stand-in for a foetus.

The juxtaposition of the Wellcome Disease Woman in the same opening as the schematic Nine-Figure Series diagrams demonstrates the only attempt to reconcile the esoteric abstraction of these twelfth-century anatomical images with the increasing prioritization of the physical experience, requiring more naturalism and the body itself to communicate these ideas.[20] The Wellcome Disease Woman is still mostly comprised of words rather than anatomy; the importance of the female, defined by her role in reproduction, was difficult to communicate solely through image. But the figure was evidently effective and popular, both for treatment and as an art object. Unlike the abstracted

hec est tertia figura
anothomie in qua de-
muntur mat's et cv°
nctuli et in qua par
te iacet et hec designa
in ne ar editur q° possit
ascedc usq: ad diafra
gma nec inouer sufoca
tom sicut·e·multas ro
nes asiguat ut inocre
maistre potentis in hoc
libro notabiliu de uui
oribus·

32 *Figura* 10: Female body featuring the seven-celled uterus, from Guido of Vigevano, *Anatomia Philippi septimi* (1345).

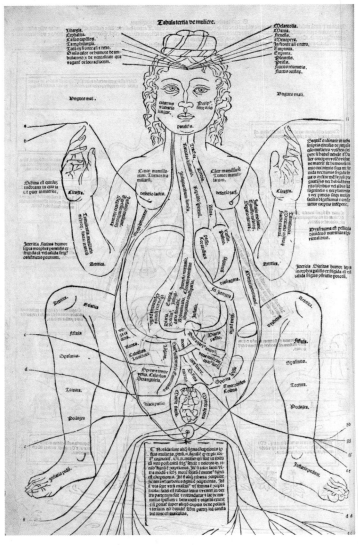

33 Disease Woman, woodcut from *Fasciculus medicinae* (1491).

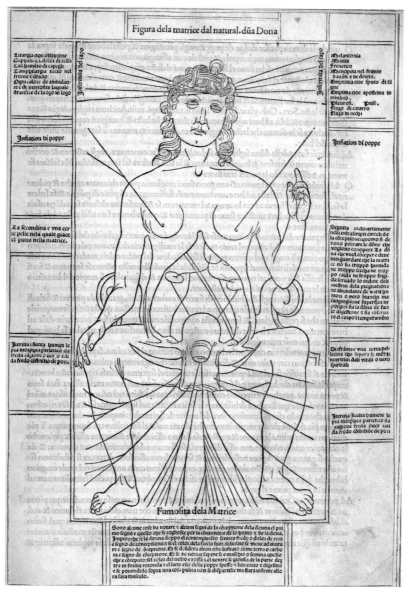

34 Disease Woman, woodcut from *Fasciculo de medicina* (1493/4).

organ diagrams or the Five-Figure Series, the Disease Woman was one of the few medieval anatomical diagrams to make it into print; it was included in the popular *Fasciculus medicinae* ('little bundle' of medicine), first printed in 1491 (illus. 33). In it, she is pictured with a bulging abdomen, unrealistically large to accommodate the description, owing in large part to her hand-drawn medieval predecessors; but the first Italian edition of 1493/4 (illus. 34) would see her relaxed to a more classicized and realistic shape, conforming with the increasing desire for perfected verisimilitude in art and medicine. While the Disease Woman is not explicitly an astrological diagram, the figure still fits with the later medieval emphasis on full-body figures that united practical and theoretical medicine to help a physician in diagnosing and treating patients; an important aspect of this was the astrological implications that had to be considered during treatment.

* * *

The types of images discussed in this chapter provided their users with information on exterior factors that would affect the functioning of the interior. The use of the full-body figure placed the practice of surgical and therapeutic interventions on the canvas of the body, relatable to the viewer and acting as a map for the practitioner. As was the case with the anatomical diagrams discussed in Chapter One, they relied on textual captions and descriptions within and around the images to further explicate complicated medical theories. Although most zodiac, bloodletting and disease figures did not include visualizations of the internal organs, those that did explicitly linked the hidden interior with the universe, reinforcing the belief that each person was connected to far greater forces than themselves and imbuing the functioning of an individual's body with a larger significance than just the mundane aches and pains of the flesh.

PART II

ANATOMY AND SURGERY

ture ou auſſ come une laugue ſem
blable a eſplam de pore ſi com dit
le phioſophe en·iz·deſ hyſtoures·
Zirbus·⁊·rebuche du zirbus
eſt membre oſſical compoſt
de veines et dartores les quelles
nourriſſent ⁊ vuniſient la tunique qui
eſt par dehors du ſtomach de la quel
tunique zirbus deſpent·les veines
⁊ les artores qui iluec ſe tiſſeut en
ſemble auſqueles le ſanc meſtru eſt
cler eſt aiouſtee ⁊ lequel ſanc eſt co
aguile p froidure et de ce eſt couerte
zirbus omentu lacharnoſite du ſto
mach et du ventre eſt tout un·et·z·
vtilites ſont de la creation du zirbus
⁊ La·i· qui deſſende en aucune ma
niere les membres nutritis deſ muiſe
ment dehors ⁊ La·2· que il a forſe
et conforte la digeſtion de tous les
membres nutritis par ſon eſpir
ſere ⁊ li̇ʒe zirbe depent du ſtomach,
due au parail ⁊ auronne tous les
membres nutritis qui ſont dedens
⁊ le zirbe tel eſt tant ſeulement
en home ceſt a ſauoir dedens le cuer
et environ a ce que la digeſtion de
lui ſont conforcee ⁊ le quiel eſt en
lui plus feible que es autres beſtes·
⁊ pour·2· choſes ⁊ La·i· car il a le
cuir du ventre tenue ⁊ La·2· en
il na paſ le ventre pelu com les au
tres beſtes·La·23· rebuche de la na
thome de la maitrique deſ reins ⁊ de
la veſſie·et deſ parties dicoiſ com
⁊·iz· figure qui eſt deuiſe par
enbas la moitie dun home
deſ la iointure de leſpine qui eſt ou
mihen deſ coſtes due au iointures
deſ pieſ contre par le mihen deſ la
ſource du ventre due au cul en la
quele apert longation geſant

ſuſ leſpine et ſus les reins ioute
les coſtes de leſpine ⁊ les porreſ vn
tiques venant a euls de la veine lu
li·et paſſans dens a la veſſie et la
veſſie entiere·et le vit trenchie par
le mihen et la coille et les coillons
entiers dont lun aparra en lune
partie de la coille et lautre en lautre

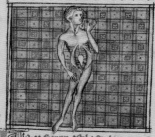

⁊a·iz· figure eſt la ſeule moitie
deſſus de ſame deſ la iointu
re de leſpine qui eſt ou mihen deſ
coſtes due aus doiſ deſ piez trenchie
par le mihen du ventre de la ſourſe
du ſtomach due au cul en la quele
apert lanuatrique geſant ſus
le longation· et les·2· coillant de
deus lie entre le col delie et la grāt
concamite· et apert la veſſie eſtā
ſut le col delie dedens entre les quā
dilles de la queue et les oſ deſ han
ches·

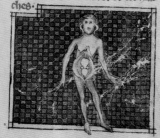

35 Dissected figures, from Henry of Mondeville, *Chirurgia* (1314).

THREE

Cutting Cadavers: Surgeons, Anatomy and the Establishment of Human Dissection

In 1304, medical students at the University of Montpellier were presented with an unusual teaching aid by their master, Henry of Mondeville (c. 1260–1320): models of individual organs to help them gain a clearer idea of the shape, size and properties of each.[1] While the original models do not survive, drawings made in the margins of copies of his works, perhaps by his students as they sat in his lectures, give us a general sense of what they might have looked like: basic line sketches of organs such as the heart and womb, and several views of the skull.[2] They do not attempt to communicate as much information as the schematic diagrams of the Nine-Figure Series, but rather depict the organs as simplified versions of what appears in life.

Henry subsequently decided to try using a graphic approach similar to the Five-Figure Series a few years later, supplementing his lectures at the University of Paris with full-body figures, drawings of which can be seen in illustrations 35, 39 and 40. Although these are not as organized or informative as the Five-Figure Series – there are no helpful captions describing the organs or their functions, and their exposed internal organs are simple, vague outlines – Henry's choice to include visual aids while teaching anatomy represents one of the most important turning points in the history of anatomy and surgery. The surgeon explained the

presence of images in his *Anatomia* (Anatomy) as the means 'by
which alone the entire anatomy and inquiry into the human
body . . . and each of its members, internal and external, in whole
and in part . . . can be demonstrated with great precision'.[3] He
further describes the usefulness of teaching with the help of
three-dimensional models:

> Anyone who wants to demonstrate the anatomy of the
> head inside and out, perfectly and in detail, should – if he
> cannot obtain a real human head – employ an artificial
> skull that can be opened, serrated to show the commissures,
> and separable into four parts so that after he has demon-
> strated its external anatomy he can open it and let the
> anatomy of the pannicles and brain be seen in detail.
> Such a skull ought to be furnished on the outside with
> things to represent the hair, the skin, the muscles, and
> the pericranium; inside it there should be something to
> represent in detail the form of the pannicles and the brain.[4]

These instructions on how to make a model of a skull reveal
Henry's conviction that his students needed to see the complicated structures of the interior to understand them, rather than
merely read or hear about them. Furthermore, he prioritized
exterior and interior views that mimicked nature, rather than
an abstracted diagram that could communicate more concepts
at the expense of reality, as in the Nine-Figure Series brain diagram (see illus. 19). His justification of the usefulness of figures
and models is the first defence of visual learning in medieval
anatomy (save, perhaps, for the inclusion of 'The picture says
the rest' in the Cambridge manuscript). Henry was the first medieval medical practitioner to acknowledge that reading lengthy
descriptions of physiology was not as effective as reading lengthy
descriptions of physiology with the help of images. The form of

his images also portended the growing desire for representation of anatomy as it appears in life, which, I argue, can be directly linked to the establishment of human dissection as a part of medical curricula around 1300.

The images discussed in the previous chapters circulated through monastic, private devotional and practical medical contexts as anonymously created, explanatory figures that united word and graphics to create a single representation of different medical theories. These diagrams could (and did) stand on their own without further need for prose explication. The establishment of medicine as a subject of university study would fundamentally change the composition and use of anatomical diagrams. In addition to the translation and dissemination of new anatomical texts, educated surgeons began to compose their own anatomical descriptions as part of their original surgical manuals, which united practical technique with theoretical physiology.[5] Anatomy was considered a crucial component to the study of surgery, and would lead to Mondino dei Liuzzi's composition of his own guide to anatomy organized as a handbook for human dissection, the *Anathomia* of 1316/17.

While these manuals were initially unillustrated, Henry of Mondeville chose to break with the text-based precedent of his teachers and contemporaries. What inspired him to become the first known creator of anatomical images in medieval Europe? Why did he create his images as two- and three-dimensional classroom models, and what role did he play in their actual composition and reproduction in manuscript form? In order to understand his motivations and those of subsequent surgical authors who also created anatomical images, it is necessary to go back to the establishment of surgery as a theoretical subject, rather than simply a manual craft learned through apprenticing. Integral, too, is the introduction of human dissection as a component of medical curricula.

Both of these crucial developments occurred at or around the University of Bologna. It was there that human dissection was first mentioned as taking place as early as 1275. Although not actually documented until 1315, when Mondino dei Liuzzi described performing two dissections of female corpses, his mention of the practice is so matter of fact that it seems it was already a well-established 'extra-curricular' activity by that point.[6] As a student at Bologna in the 1280s and 1290s, Henry of Mondeville most likely witnessed human dissections. But the practice was slow to spread elsewhere, including to the universities of Montpellier and Paris where Henry subsequently taught, and so he chose to give his students the best stand-in that he could in the form of models and figures. This chapter will explore the variety of components that led to the establishment of human dissection at the University of Bologna and its effect on anatomical teaching and learning in general, and on the development of Henry's figures more specifically.[7]

The Rise of University Surgery

Although we know medicine was taught in Salerno well before it is documented anywhere else, medical faculties in universities in general remained amorphous and unregulated for some time: there were neither formal guidelines stating what must be taught and by whom, nor a process for granting a recognized degree certifying the graduate had attained a certain level of training. Around the year 1200, as universities were forming across Europe, medical education began to take shape: masters gathered cohorts of students, established which texts were most important to teach and decided at what point their students had learned enough to take a degree and begin teaching themselves. Medical faculties provided protections for educated physicians and, in turn, allowed them to both regulate and establish standards for those claiming proficiency in the field. Although many factors led to the transformation of medicine from a manual skill to a university-recognized *scientia* (a subject that could be ordered by reason and was therefore able to be taught), the spread and assimilation of Aristotelian philosophy into medical practice contributed. Also, the growing influence of regulations based on classical Roman laws led to the establishment of guilds and legal standards within communities. European cities came to rely on university-trained physicians for advice during out-breaks of disease – most notably seen in the Black Death pandemic of the mid-fourteenth century – and eventually established pro-fessional licensing systems that were intended to protect patients from charlatans.

Surgery was not immediately taught in early medical faculties. Like medicine in general, surgery was traditionally a craft passed from master to student, often within the same family, unencum-bered by the need for literacy or academic study and focused instead on technical skills. Practitioners had to know the basics of human anatomy to successfully perform their crafts: the barber understood how the bones fit together to set breaks, the apothecary where to find a vein for bloodletting and the midwife the shape of the uterus and vaginal canal.[8] Most early practition-ers performed life-saving measures or standard physical interven-tions (like tooth extraction) that did not require an in-depth understanding of Galenic medical or physiological theory.[9] Two of the most common surgical procedures were cautery and bloodletting, relatively non-invasive techniques that were not only prophylactic but performed to restore humoral harmony. More serious surgeries were treatments of traumas, like dressing and stitching wounds, setting fractures, dislocations and broken bones, removing foreign objects from the body, amputation and even rare instances of trepanning, drilling a hole into the skull to relieve pressure on the brain. Some of the most famous images of medieval surgery feature a surgeon treating a head wound – removing pieces of the skull and bandaging the injury – below scenes from Christ's life (British Library, Sloane MS 1977; illus. 36). The images accompany a copy of what is considered to be the first 'academic' surgical manual written in Latin, the *Chirurgia* (Surgery) of Roger Frugardi (*fl.* 1170).[10] Roger's treatise differs from other surgical texts of the time, which were mostly presented as a list of procedures according to body parts, because it provides a prose explanation of the types of ailments that required treatment by surgeons, thereby defining the discipline. Roger provides a description of the process of diagnosis and step-by-step instructions for treatments. While it would be surpassed by more innovative and advanced manuals, Roger's *Chirurgia* remained popular throughout the Middle Ages, appearing in vernacular translations across Europe. Sloane MS 1977 is a richly illuminated French version of his treatise made some two and a half centuries after it was first written. The juxtaposition between the Christological cycle and images of surgical treatment might have served as a reminder to the viewer that while surgeons and medical practitioners did the best that they could to save the living, Christ was considered the ultimate healer for both the body and the soul.[11]

As medical faculties began to establish themselves, so too did literate surgeons, keen to distinguish their art from that of uneducated barbers by promoting surgery as an important aspect of medical knowledge, worthy of university study. Known as the 'rational' surgeons, these educated practitioners incorporated Galenic theory into their surgical manuals.[12] While initially confined to the early medical faculties around the Mediterranean, rational surgery spread to Paris by the late thirteenth century via the establishment of the College of St Cosmas, an independent educational institution begun by learned surgeons when the University of Paris refused to recognize surgery as a discipline.[13]

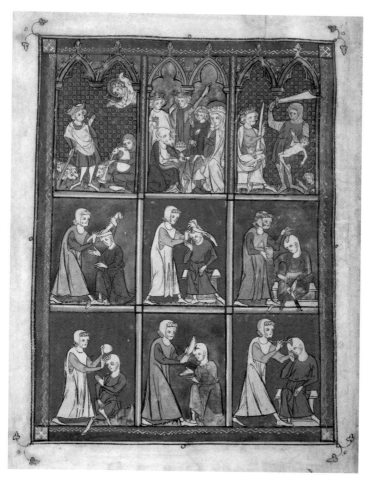

36 Scenes from Christ's life (top register), above scenes from the operation on a compound skull fracture (bottom two registers), from Roger Frugardi, *Chirurgia* (c. 1300–1325).

Rational surgery was slower to spread to northern Europe; the universities at Oxford and Cambridge had no surgical faculties, and the first documented university-trained surgeons in England did not appear until the fourteenth century.[14]

The general overviews of anatomy included in the most widespread and influential medical texts of the Middle Ages, most especially Constantine the African's *Pantegni* and the late twelfth-century translation of Avicenna's *Al-Qānūn fī al-ṭibb* (*Canon of Medicine*), continued to reign as the most common anatomical texts. But the rational surgeons took Galen's exhortation of the importance of anatomy to heart, including a section devoted to the subject in their surgical manuals. The earliest 'new' anatomical treatise attributed to a European author was written by William of Saliceto (*c.* 1210–1277), a surgeon who trained in Bologna and devoted an entire book of his *Chirurgia* (revised version finished in 1275) to the subject. William and subsequent rational surgeons – relying upon the *Pantegni* and other Galenic works – quoted Galen's insistence on knowledge of anatomy, specifically through dissection, as crucial to understanding the workings of the body.[15] His student Lanfranc of Milan (*c.* 1250–1306) was responsible for bringing Italian surgical training to Paris in the 1290s. Although William was the first to have a discrete anatomical section, it was Lanfranc who placed it at the very beginning of his own work, completed in 1296. He explained (quoting William almost exactly) that Galen believed a surgeon must understand anatomy – meaning both the situation of the organs within the body as well as their functions and complexions – before he could truly recognize on which part he should operate:

> Since, as Galen says, it is necessary for a surgeon to know the anatomy, so that he does not think that an extended ligament is skin, or that a round-shaped ligament is a nerve, or plunge into his operations in error, I have represented the natures and forms of the parts of the body, remedies for them, and their complexions.[16]

The fundamental structures of the body – ligaments, muscles, nerves – had to be understood before one could appreciate the ways in which the body operates, and subsequently devise treatments appropriate to restoring the body to its normal functions. The surgeon was just as much required to know anatomy as the physician, lest he make a mistake when cutting. The language echoes the summary of Galen's words in the anonymous *Historia incisionis*, but instead of serving as a vague warning for all physicians against erring accidentally, Lanfranc and William argue it is especially crucial for surgeons in their craft to understand the positions and properties of the interior. By 'claiming' anatomy as their remit, these rational surgeons made efforts to elevate anatomy along with surgery in university-taught medicine.

By the mid-thirteenth century, Montpellier had emerged as the foremost medical school in Europe.[17] Masters read aloud from texts recognized as fundamental to medical learning. Medical curricula differed by institution and evolved considerably between the twelfth and fifteenth centuries, but all were text-based, a set group of core treatises arranged around the foundational *Articella*. In Paris, students studied an arts curriculum as undergraduates, where they would master the natural philosophy of Aristotle, and only then were they allowed to undertake the study of medicine as graduate students. According to the requirements for a medical degree drawn up circa 1270–74 for the University of Paris, just a few decades before Henry of Mondeville would lecture there with his models, each student was supervised by a master, and in order to receive his degree in medicine, the master would have to swear to the university chancellor that the student (already possessing a Bachelor of Arts) had attended lectures on the required texts for at least five and a half years. In addition to the *Articella*, these texts included Constantine's *Viaticum* and the *Antidotary*, a collection of practical remedies written in Salerno by a master known only as Nicholas in the late twelfth century.[18] At the University of Bologna, undergraduate students could go right into the medical curriculum, studying it and the arts at the same time. Taddeo Alderotti (d. 1295) carefully crafted the medical curriculum there to be both practical and theoretical.[19] He began teaching after establishing a successful medical practice and emphasized the importance of mastering the foundational arts and fundamental medical works and, under his guidance, the first provision requiring an annual demonstration of human dissection was implemented around 1275.

Anatomy and Dissection in Medical Curricula

How did the idea to include dissection in university medical curricula first arise? Taddeo's inclusion of the process as part of the course of study at the University of Bologna is both radical and mundane: radical because it is the first reference to university cadaveric dissection in the Middle Ages, and mundane because there is little evidence it caused much of a stir, since there are no contemporary mentions of such demonstrations actually occurring. Either they were so uneventful as to be entirely absent from records, or they did not happen at all. But the fact that Taddeo included a provision for dissection in his curriculum demonstrates how human dissection fit into medieval medical learning. Contrary to the persistent myth that the Church forbade human dissection in the Middle Ages,[20] it was in fact a learning tool devised and developed by medieval thinkers and not simply a resurrection of a classical practice.[21]

A precursor to the establishment of human dissection is the evidence of pig dissections being performed as early as the twelfth century, attested to by a series of texts known as the Salernitan Demonstrations.[22] Possibly composed in Salerno (although this is not certain), the texts guide a dissector through the anatomy of a pig and clearly demonstrate the influence of Constantine the African's *Pantegni*, which represented the most advanced anatomical knowledge at the time. However, the Demonstrations do not explain *why* such experiments were considered a worthwhile complement to the study of medicine. This indicates that anatomy was an acceptable field of study because of the insistences of Galen and his Islamic consolidators, but not necessarily unto itself; ultimately, it seems these dissections did not affect the study of diseases and treatments in any significant way, nor were they considered integral to medical understanding. That said, the remarkable fact that pig dissections were occurring over the course of several centuries establishes an awareness of the visual benefits of conducting dissections on an animal known to have a similar interior to humans. That the texts are in dialogue with each other, as subsequent physicians disagreed with previous versions of the text and added their own instructions, further indicates a thriving practice in southern Italy.[23] However, there is no evidence such experiments happened outside of Salerno. We must look to evidence beyond medical learning to see the different ways bodies were being opened with increasing frequency in medieval culture, paving the way for human dissection.[24]

The twelfth century saw the rediscovery of Greek and Roman legal texts in Italy, which affected the establishment of civil legal systems in towns and the formation of faculties of law in universities (especially Bologna), and led to the earliest autopsy examinations held to determine the causes of suspicious deaths. In the papal decretals of 1209, it is recorded that Pope Innocent III (1160–1216) ordered two post-mortems be conducted on people believed to have been poisoned, the findings of which were used as evidentiary bases for papal rulings.[25] This suggests that as early as the first decade of the thirteenth century, autopsy was not only accepted but sought out to determine causes of death, and coroners' findings were trusted as admissible evidence even in the highest court in medieval Europe.

Visual evidence attests to the presence of autopsies as early as the thirteenth century in two manuscripts made at opposite ends of Europe: England and Spain. They are the only known pre-1300 manuscript depictions of autopsies and, notably, both corpses are female.[26] The first is from a miniature cycle in the English MS Ashmole 399 (discussed previously for the Nine-Figure Series content), bound in circa 1298 or 1299 (illus. 20–22). The series of eight scenes on a discrete bifolium depicting the illness, death and graphic autopsy (illus. 37) of a woman was inserted seemingly at random in the middle of Constantine the African's translation of a treatise on the stomach. Dated to the second half of the thirteenth century on stylistic grounds – the miniatures reflect popular designs found in mid- to late thirteenth-century English manuscript illumination – the first four miniatures include banderoles (speech scrolls) that were likely meant to include text but were never filled in, leaving later viewers to guess at the narrative and source. The final two scenes were added by a different hand and feature a line of women complaining of different disorders and hoping to be treated by a physician, potentially illustrating a text attributed to a female physician, Trota of Salerno (fl. c. 1100–1150), on cosmetics.[27]

The autopsy miniature is striking. A female corpse lies prostrate, hair unbound and flowing, breasts and skin shrivelled, cut open from breastbone to pubic bone. Her organs – red and brown kidneys, blue lungs, red and pink heart – float in mid-air around her body. A barber-surgeon standing at her feet holds her liver in one hand and his upraised knife in the other, facing the physician, gowned and capped, who points to the corpse. The physician is presumably instructing the barber-surgeon, the manual labourer, on how to proceed. He is shadowed by a hooded assistant. This scene is significant for many reasons, not the least of which is the rarity of the practice of autopsy, especially on women, at the time. The association of women with purity, chastity and weakness meant that the exposure of a woman's naked body to anyone not her husband or family,

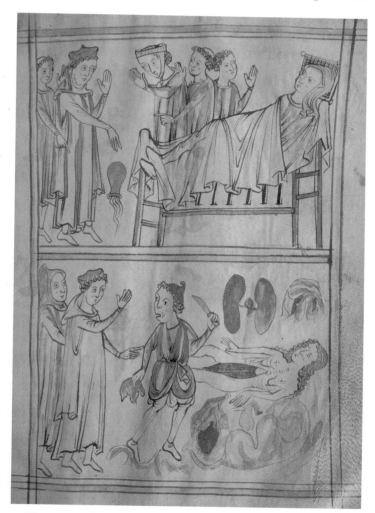

37 Woman undergoing treatment by physician (top), and autopsy (bottom), from *Miscellanea medica* [England] (c. 1250–1310).

even in death, would only have been undertaken in remarkable circumstances. Most likely, the Ashmole cycle depicts a wealthy woman who died so suddenly that poisoning of some nature was supposed, and her family subsequently requested a post-mortem examination to discover material proof.[28]

The second image of a female autopsy, roughly contemporary with the Ashmole 399 image, is overtly religious in nature. A richly illuminated copy of the *Cantigas de Santa María* (Songs of Saint Mary) known as the 'Codicé rico', made at the court of Alfonso x the Wise, king of Castile and León, between 1280 and 1284, includes a song that recounts a young woman's heart being cut open following her sudden death (illus. 38) to determine if she was poisoned.[29] Illustrated in detail across six scenes, Cantiga 188 describes the young woman as so devoted to the Virgin Mary that she found she could no longer live in this world. She chose to stop eating and grew very ill. On her deathbed, the song says, whenever her distraught family mentioned the Virgin, she would gesture wordlessly to her heart. Her parents suspected that she had been poisoned, and when she finally succumbed, they had her heart cut open to look for evidence; instead, they found an image of the Virgin engraved in her flesh. The fifth miniature depicts this post-mortem in detail: her family surrounds her bedside while an otherwise unidentified man holds a knife in her heart. According to the song, her family immediately went to offer their prayers and thanksgiving to the Virgin Mary for the physical evidence of her presence in their daughter.

The fact that the woman's family in Cantiga 188 requested her heart be cut open, and that the Ashmole miniature takes care to depict the involvement of family members in the illness, treatment and death of the woman, reinforces the acceptance of autopsy during the thirteenth century as a means to determine cause of death in remarkable or suspicious circumstances. While poisoning was suspected in the case of the *Cantigas* woman and it turns out to be a miraculous sign of the Virgin's favour, her story clearly prefigures those of the Italian holy women Chiara of Montefalco (d. 1308) and Margarita of Città di Castello (d. 1320) a few decades later, whose hearts were also opened following long illnesses and similar complaints of chest pain.

In Chiara's case, her fellow nuns found symbols of the Passion, including a crucifix and a scourge, within her heart, as well as three stones in her gallbladder.[30] In contrast, the *Cantigas* woman's story is anonymous; there are no hints about her identity beyond that she was from a wealthy family. In the absence of other clues for now, we may make a few deductions. The *Cantigas* were compiled at Alfonso's behest and with his direct involvement, and many of the songs recounting miracles describe local details, including the city in which each holy event is alleged to have happened.[31] Cantiga 188 is given no such identifying features, and so it is possible, if not probable, that the story came from outside of Alfonso's realm, and so can perhaps be connected to the Italian autopsies or even the Ashmole narrative.

The existence of these images and accounts of autopsy are indicative of the broader changing nature of the relationship between medicine and the body in the thirteenth century.

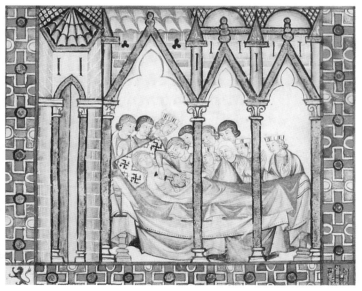

38 Post-mortem of young woman's heart, detail from Cantiga 188 of the *Cantigas de Santa María* (1280–84).

Coinciding with the influx of new Aristotelian and Galenic texts translated from the Middle East and assimilated into medieval culture in the twelfth and thirteenth centuries – especially those asserting the importance of empirical observation (and Galen's particular exhortation of the importance of physical examination of the body) – they demonstrate a movement toward a more hands-on approach to the body previously felt to be unnecessary. The first recorded public opening of the body since antiquity occurred in Bologna in 1302: the autopsy of the criminal Azzolino, as part of a judicial proceeding to determine if Azzolino had been poisoned.[32] The University of Bologna was famed for its large and influential legal faculty alongside its faculty of medicine, and it is no coincidence that the first public autopsy ordered by a judge took place in that city. The development of dissection should thus be seen as not a new break with convention, but rather as an organic extension of a developing practice rooted in both Church and municipal law.[33]

Dissection in Bologna

The historical epithet 'restorer of anatomy' was bestowed on surgeon Mondino dei Liuzzi because his popular anatomical text – the *Anathomia* – was structured from the perspective of one performing a human dissection, and fundamentally altered the way anatomical treatises were composed.[34] Born into the wealthy Florentine Liuzzi family around 1265, Mondino came from a medical clan; his father was an apothecary and his uncle taught medicine at the University of Bologna. Mondino followed in his uncle's footsteps, studying under Taddeo Alderotti and spending the rest of his life teaching medicine and anatomy at the university. Mondino chose to organize his *Anathomia*, which was likely composed over several years and finished no earlier than 1316, as a series of step-by-step instructions for dissecting a corpse, into which he wove descriptions of Galenic physiology. Mondino's treatise became the most well-known anatomical text of the later Middle Ages, circulating in manuscript and then in printed form well into the sixteenth century. Although Mondino did not personally have his manual illustrated, later copies of the work sometimes were (see, for instance, illus. 65 and 71).

Mondino places the reader in the position of dissector from the outset, framing his description of the body as if standing before a corpse on a dissecting table: 'Having laid out the body of one that has died from beheading or hanging in the supine position, we must first gain an idea of the whole, and secondly, of the parts.'[35] He furthermore does not organize his discussion by the 'simple' (what he deems 'similar') and 'complex' ('composite') parts, as the earlier *Historia incisionis* and Nine-Figure Series were, for the pragmatic reason that it is not possible to see the simple parts (veins, arteries, bones, nerves and muscles) easily in the course of performing a dissection. As he puts it: 'Although there are two kinds of parts, similar and composite, I shall not make a separate anatomy of those that are similar, for their anatomy is not fully visible in a body which has been cut up, but rather in one decomposed in streams of water.'[36] Leaving aside the possibility that he put bodies in streams to decompose, Mondino's text proposed a new way to approach human anatomy, one based on the practicalities of dissecting a cadaver. He divided the body into three 'venters', or cavities – the abdomen, chest and skull – and began his text with the abdomen 'because the organs there smell bad and therefore I shall begin with them so they can be discarded first'.[37] Notably, the first organ he discusses in the 'lower venter' is the uterus. He explains he dissected two women the year before, one in January and one in March, and so has seen the uterus in detail. However, in the course of his description of the female reproductive system, he reiterates the anatomically incorrect Galenic argument that the uterus contains seven compartments. His repetition of the myth of the seven-celled uterus demonstrates the dominance of authoritative texts despite his own experiments. Whether he saw seven compartments in the uterus(es) he dissected or not, he chose to espouse the idea in his treatise.

Despite Mondino's casual mention of the multiple dissections he was able to undertake in a single year, implying they happened regularly at the University of Bologna, there is little to indicate they occurred elsewhere with such frequency. The practice spread slowly, first to other northern Italian universities, then to Montpellier and beyond over the course of the fourteenth and fifteenth centuries. University statutes reveal that even though dissection was included in medical curricula, there is no evidence that they happened as regularly as stated, if indeed they happened at all. For example, statutes written for the medical school at Montpellier in the 1340s stipulate a dissection must be held once every two years, but we have no contemporary documents corroborating their occurrence.[38] The University of Bologna statutes of 1405, which are the earliest complete records of the medical curriculum there, detail the ways in which a body could be procured for the annual dissection (usually, it had to be an executed criminal from outside the city whose body went unclaimed by their family), how many students were allowed to attend (more for a female corpse than a male; presumably, a rarer occurrence) and the fees incurred by the students and university to put on the dissection.[39] Evidence of dissections happening in northern Europe, especially Germany, England and France, before the late fifteenth century is also scarce.[40]

The slow spread of the practice can be attributed to the fact that dissection was a messy and costly procedure that was not deemed wholly necessary to medical education. Medieval scholars believed Galen performed human and animal dissection (although he only ever dissected the latter), and faith in Galen's reliability meant it was not considered necessary to repeat his experiments to 'check' if he was correct, but rather to imitate his process to demonstrate his points to students. Debates and theoretical dissections of authoritative texts were the major ways in which physiological issues were discussed, and a dissected corpse was not very useful in that sense. Any disconnect between medical authorities – the most prominent example being differences between Aristotle and Galen's opinions on physiology and anatomy – were debated in the classroom.[41]

Henry of Mondeville and Mondino dei Liuzzi: Dissection and Image

Henry of Mondeville and his visual aids were roughly contemporary with Mondino dei Liuzzi's anatomical text, and Henry's work demonstrates the influence of Bolognese surgical and anatomical teaching in which he was trained. His *Chirurgia*, written in 1306 and subsequently revised and updated until his death in 1320, begins with a section dedicated to anatomy. Following Mondino's lead, Henry divided his anatomical section so that it emphasized the compound members over the simple members, proceeding according to the three venters in the order Mondino described, beginning with the abdomen, followed by the thorax and ending with the skull. Since Mondino and Henry were contemporaries, and Henry began writing his treatise around the same time as Mondino, it is likely that both men modelled their surgical texts after what was common practice in Bologna. Mondino's would circulate much more widely, however, and so he is credited with the innovative format.

But Mondino did not include images in his texts, nor do we have references to him teaching with the help of visual aids. Indeed, it is possible that Henry's incorporation of images was not looked upon favourably by his contemporaries because there was a preference for dissections over reproductions of dissected corpses. Guy of Chauliac, who achieved fame with his own surgical text (the *Chirurgia magna* of 1363) that included a linear history of the surgeons who worked at Bologna, disagreed with Henry's inclusion of images, arguing that Galen learned through dissecting: 'And by these methods [dissections] did Galen notice these things in the bodies of humans and apes, and not through pictures – as the previously mentioned Henry [of Mondeville] has done, who has been seen teaching anatomy with thirteen pictures.'[42] Guy implies that Henry's images were a poor substitute for first-hand explorations and should not be used as a crutch.

While we cannot be certain of the exact appearance of the 'thirteen pictures' to which Guy refers, there are several different types of images associated with Henry. A manuscript that allegedly reproduces the simple organ models Henry taught with in Montpellier in 1304 depicts them as pen sketches either in the margins or incorporated into text columns.[43] In this and two slightly later witnesses, the figures are workaday: functional, small and uncoloured, labelled with a word or two. The organs drawn include the skull and its sutures, the heart, the liver, the gallbladder, the spleen, the kidneys and the bladder. There are also images of an 'empty' and 'full' uterus, although there is no foetus pictured.

Supposed copies of the full-length figures devised by Henry to accompany his lectures in Paris in 1306 are found in two extant manuscripts: one a gilded French translation of 1314 (Paris, Bibliothèque nationale de France, MS fr. 2030; see illus. 35),[44] and one a simple Latin copy, dated to the fourteenth century (Trinity College, Cambridge, MS O.2.44; illus. 39, 40).[45] There is no indication Henry was aware of the older Five-Figure Series when creating his full-body images. In addition to depicting systems like the skeleton and muscles frontally, Henry introduced a dorsal

viewpoint: the skeleton and figures showing the organs of the
thorax and abdomen are pictured from the back as well. The
dorsal skeletons do not resemble the dorsal tradition associated
with Islamic anatomical images of the late fourteenth century,
but rather indicate the influence of popular contemporary 'Dance
of Death' skeletons (see illus. 58), macabre and grinning, a stark
contrast to the gentle fleshy bone figures of the Five-Figure
Series.[46] In each of Henry's full-body figures, the bodies are living and in motion, gesturing to their insides or holding their skins
over their shoulders like the flayed saint Bartholomew. By presenting the anatomy of living bodies, Henry reminds the viewer
that the point of dissection was for students to understand what
a healthy, alive body ought to look like, and so be able to recognize abnormal signs of illness and disease in order to treat their
patients.[47]

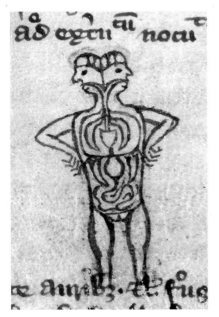 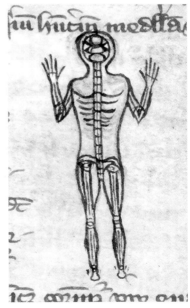

39, 40 Frontal bisected figure and dorsal skeleton, from Henry of Mondeville,
Chirurgia (early 14th century).

BnF MS fr. 2030, the French vernacular version of Henry's *Chirurgia*, was produced in Paris and features animated, energetic dissected bodies in column-width miniatures. The manuscript begins with a full-page miniature that appears to depict Henry instructing a group of students. Henry, or another physician, is only present in two of the thirteen images; otherwise, the dissected bodies are solo. The use of colour and luxurious gold leaf throughout indicate it was an expensive production, perhaps made for Henry's royal patrons: he became surgeon to the French kings Philip IV (1268–1314) and Louis X (1289–1316) in Paris before his death in 1320. BnF MS fr. 2030 stands in stark contrast to the line sketches of the Trinity manuscript, drawn by an amateur artist, with no luxurious accents.[48] None of Henry's full-body figures include labels, but the existence of each image is noted in the text by number, serving as chapter divisions. In BnF MS fr. 2030, these captions appear directly beside each figure, while some hunting for each reference is required in the Trinity version.

Although an early twentieth-century historian proclaimed these small drawings to be unskilled and rudimentary copies of what they assumed were the far more detailed models and figures actually used by Henry in his lectures, there is in fact no indication that the figures are simplified. Rather, they provide a general overview of what one might view inside the opened human body without any real emphasis on the specific form of the organs. This was, after all, not the point of the figures. Instead, they were designed to relay an overall sense of a dissected corpse; the textual explications of Henry's writing were tasked with providing details. The images are an indication of the changing nature of graphics in academic learning: useful as general guides and more practically as a way to break up a text, but not trying to encompass layers of teleological information. They also indicate the rising emphasis on seeing the interior, as Galen exhorted. Henry chose to help his students visualize it with (stench-free, easily manipulated) images at a time when actual human dissections remained rare.

* * *

While it is certainly true that most early dissections were undertaken only as a visual demonstration of established theories, the tendency in modern scholarship to dismiss all medieval human dissections as derivative and uncurious is misleading. The educated surgeons discussed in this chapter sometimes took issue with Galen's and Avicenna's arguments, drawing upon what they saw within the body during their own dissections as evidence for refuting their claims.

Other than the record provided by Guy of Chauliac, which simply attests to Henry of Mondeville's use of figures in the course of his teaching, we do not know the details of how much input Henry had in the actual composition of the images he used. We can infer from his writings that he clearly felt they were useful, and he describes in detail what models (like the skull) should include. But we have no record that he collaborated with an artist or workshop to produce his models and figures, nor do we know if he exerted any control over the way they were copied in the lavish manuscript made during his lifetime (BnF MS fr. 2030). Another student of Bologna, Guido of Vigevano, working some three decades after Henry's death, would take his appreciation of visual aids to the next level.

FOUR

Fourteenth-Century Anatomical Images, Latin West and Islamic Middle East

Aside from the Italian artist Leonardo da Vinci, the Flemish anatomist Andreas Vesalius springs to mind most readily when considering art and anatomy before 1600. This is due in part to the traditional historiographic emphasis on the innovations of the scientific revolution, reducing medical knowledge – especially anatomical – to 'pre-Vesalian' and 'post-Vesalian'. Vesalius's monumental printed anatomical manual *De humani corporis fabrica* (*On the Fabric of the Human Body*) of 1543 catapulted him to fame in large part because of the remarkably detailed woodcut illustrations accompanying the lengthy work. The *Fabrica* was so popular that it became ubiquitous in anatomical learning and teaching, so influential that it replaced nearly all earlier works.[1] Vesalius played an active role in the composition of his images, which number more than two hundred. The frontispiece is particularly well-known: it presents a chaotic scene of dissection, featuring the author himself at the centre of the action as he teaches from an opened female corpse (illus. 41). In the image and preface to his text, Vesalius railed against the typical format of contemporary dissections, in which there was a division of labour between the lecturer, dissector and ostensor (pointer), with the learned physician professor occupying the first position, a barber-surgeon the second and a student or other instructor the third.

Although Vesalius endeavoured to position himself as a revolutionary, rebelling against the norms of his contemporaries who did not perform dissections with their own hands but rather 'squawk[ed] like jackdaws from their lofty professorial chairs things they have never done but only memorize from the books of others or see written down',[2] he was preceded by a medieval surgeon who also produced an illustrated anatomical treatise featuring images of himself performing dissections, abeit with far less influence: Guido of Vigevano, a surgeon from Lombardy who became physician to Queen Jeanne of Burgundy, wife of Philip VI (1293–1350). Like Vesalius, Guido worked with professional artists to create the full-page images that formed the central focus of his brief treatise, the *Anatomia Philippi septimi* (Anatomy for Philip VII) of 1345 (see illus. 10, 32, 42–3), and although they are comparatively smaller in number (eighteen compared to Vesalius's hundreds), the treatment of anatomical images as worthy of such prominence in a surgical manual was unprecedented.

In this chapter, we will explore Guido's unique work within the context of the anatomists and anatomical images of the thirteenth and fourteenth centuries. His insistence on the creation of and ownership over the composition of his figures would not be repeated by another surgeon until the sixteenth century.

Henry of Mondeville's Path and Guido of Vigevano

While we do not have any evidence that Henry of Mondeville worked with professional artists, his explicit acknowledgement in both his teaching and writings of the value of images must have influenced Guido, who also emerged from the teachings of the surgeons in Bologna before moving to France. Henry's use of dissected images was singular at the time, but the manuscript copies of Henry's images, including the one we know was made during his lifetime (BnF MS fr. 2030; see illus. 35), fit into the established mould for the illumination of academic texts, in

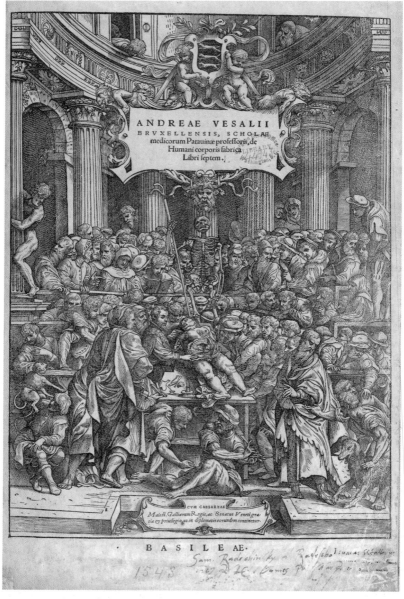

41 Dissection, frontispiece to Andreas Vesalius, *De humani corporis fabrica* (1543).

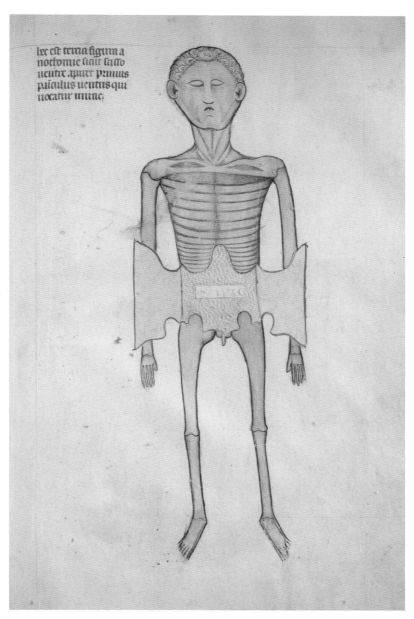

hec est tertia figura a nottomie sicut sacco uentre aperit primus pticulus uentus qui uocatur mirac

42 *Figura* 3: View of the abdominal wall, labelled *mirac*, from Guido of Vigevano, *Anatomia Philippi septimi* (1345).

which workshop artists, charged with creating imagery both useful and decorative, often used gaps in the text column or the spaces in large letters, known as historiated initials, to mark new sections in a text.

Guido wielded remarkable control over the unique and personal image cycle designed to accompany his *Anatomia*. The images only exist in one copy, which is the manuscript he evidently presented to the king, now Chantilly, Bibliothèque du musée Condé, MS 334, likely produced by professional illuminators in Paris.[3] Guido lays out his stance on the value of images as stand-ins for actual dissected bodies in the preface:

> in order that this book . . . may be more useful, [I] will plainly and openly demonstrate anatomy of the human body through illustrations, just as they are in the human body. [The anatomy] will appear in an evident fashion in the images below and rather better than it can be seen in the human body itself, because when we do the anatomy on a man, it is necessary to make haste because of the stench. Therefore doctors can only get an overall view of the inner organs, just as they lie there. Therefore, whoever wishes to see an anatomy well must see it many times, diligently, in detail, and one member after another. But since that cannot be done because the opportunities for obtaining a human body for an anatomy are rare and also because it is prohibited by the Church, I myself undertook to present an anatomy in pictures. And my qualifications to do so can be trusted, because I myself have done [anatomies] on the human body many, many times.[4]

Guido's reasons for including the images in his anatomical treatise are ostensibly to circumvent the difficulties in performing actual human dissection, but they would also have served the

more mundane purpose of aiding the viewer to remember what
he (or she, given he served the queen's household) read. Guido's
language is similar to that of William of Saliceto and Lanfranc of
Milan, among others, when he refers to 'presenting' anatomy for
his readers (Lanfranc said he 'represented the natures and forms
of the parts of the body', meaning through his text). But Guido
has gone a step further by providing images that he wished his
readers to accept as truth, just as they would Lanfranc's descriptions. Significant, though, is Guido's heavy reliance on Mondino
dei Liuzzi's writing in both his text and images. While he positions
himself as a heroic figure who has dissected many bodies and thus
should be trusted, his contribution to the history of anatomy lies
almost exclusively in the novel way in which he used images.

Of the eighteen full-page images, Guido presents himself
along with either a corpse as he dissects it (see illus. 10) or a living
patient five times; the rest are dissected corpses (or skulls) alone.
The images are colourful and skilfully drawn and include labels
or captions within the body cavities. They unite the diagrammatic tradition of the Nine-Figure Series with a narrative twist:
Guido presents himself as a solo protagonist, alone with the
cadaver, exploring its interior. But the performative undertones
of the images are as strong as those that include crowds of spectators, like in Vesalius's frontispiece. Guido's audience is the
reader, whom he hopes will be as enlightened by his images as
they would by an actual dissection, if not even more so.

The story Guido's images present – the stages of dissecting
a corpse – is slow and methodical (illus. 43). The figures proceed
according to Mondino dei Liuzzi's order, by the three venters,
with the anatomist pictured making incisions into the corpse
as the introductory figure to each new section. They demonstrate
the process of peeling back the skin in layers, revealing step by
step what one might see after each cut. Guido refers to each
image as a numbered *figura* (figure) in the short text caption to

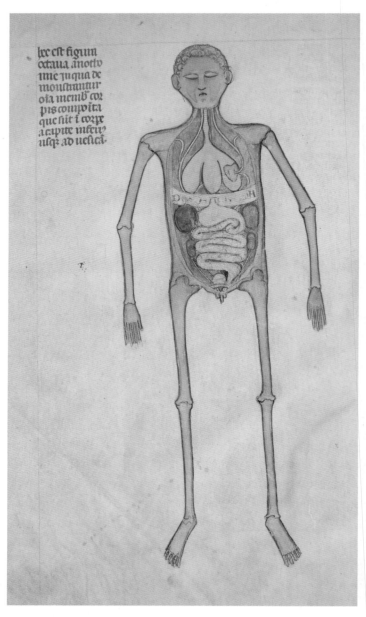

43 *Figura* 8: Organs of the abdomen and thorax, from Guido of Vigevano, *Anatomia Philippi septimi* (1345).

the left of each drawing in which he explains what they are meant to depict. While the dissected bodies discussed up until now have been living, animated bodies, aside from the first step of the dissection (featuring a living man with the names of the internal organs written on the body's surface),[5] Guido presents the viewer with what one would see at an actual anatomical dissection: corpses.[6] The bodies are greenish-grey or jaundiced, emaciated, eyes closed, and the overall effect they present is quite stylized. The limbs are long, thin and straight, the collar-bones jut out, the veins in the throats are visible. The bodies are male, evidenced by the small genitalia at the base of the torso, except for *figura* 10, which demonstrates a female corpse with a carefully proportioned seven-celled uterus (see illus. 32).

On a more practical note – and one that Vesalius also worried about – Guido describes how hard it would be for his manual to be reproduced, 'first on account of the expense, and then because it is not easy to find painters who know how to draw the figures'.[7] This is a unique recognition of the challenge of having anatomical images made, presumably as it would have been a rare request of professional illustrators, and indicates that Guido was an exacting author who took the composition of these images very seriously. Perhaps he made preparatory draw-ings himself, which a professional artist imitated and polished, or the artist brought Guido's vision to life from his descriptions. The figures reflect contemporary tropes employed by French, Italian and English artists, especially visible in the images of the skeleton, which are reminiscent of religious painting and manu-script iconography of skeletons, like works featuring the tale of the Three Living and the Three Dead.[8] Images of this moralizing tale, which describes three vain and materialistic earthly kings who confront their corpses in various states of decomposition while out riding, were fairly common; one roughly contemporary example can be found in the De Lisle Psalter, made in England

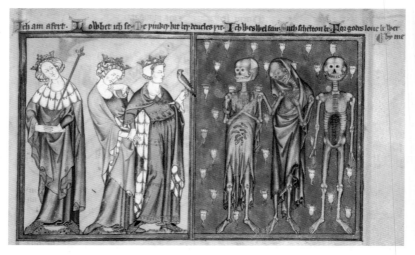

44 Legend of the Three Living and the Three Dead, from the De Lisle Psalter (c. 1310).

circa 1310 (British Library, Arundel MS 83; illus. 44).[9] Here and in Guido's images, the skeletons are thin and brittle, their joints indicated by simple jagged lines, and single bones pictured for the forearms and lower legs where, in reality, there are two bones. Their purpose is not to imitate the skeleton as it would appear in nature, but rather to create the illusion of anatomical accuracy while (in the case of the psalter) inspiring fear and revulsion in the viewer to remind them of their impending deaths.

Guido deliberately chose to have himself memorialized as an anatomist, knife in hand, revealing the mysteries of the interior to show off his expertise. His placement of himself within his illustrations portends the shift in learned anatomy from focusing on the cadaver to the person wielding the knife, which would be so effectively manipulated by Vesalius two hundred years later. But while Vesalius had access to a much wider and more receptive audience and achieved the heights of fame for his work, Guido's went largely unnoticed. There are no known copies of his images. His treatise relied on Mondino's anatomical manual, especially in his account of the process of a dissection. And despite urging his readers to witness dissections so that they can see the 'truth' of his account, his repetition (and depiction) of anatomically inaccurate traditions – like the seven-celled uterus – undermines his claims of precision and veracity.

It seems that above all Guido's aim was to create a treatise that would impress the king and queen of France with his mastery of human anatomy and experience in dissecting cadavers (which was not part of the curriculum in Paris at the time) through the accompanying figures. Guido's role as a physician in the highest court in France reveals a man interested in making a name for himself outside of university medical circles. Laymen seeking to practice medicine had the option to stay in the academic orbit, becoming teachers themselves, or to assume positions as professional healers in towns and cities across Europe. A select few, through connections or sheer ambition, were able to achieve the comfortable position of physician to nobility and royalty. These personal physicians were expected to treat all members of their patron's family, usually living in close quarters and 'on call' at all hours to regulate diet and therapeutic interventions, dress injuries and prescribe remedies for ailments.[10] Once employed by a noble or royal family, many master physicians, renowned for their learning and skills, took the opportunity to dedicate their written works to their wealthy patrons. In bringing his expertise in anatomy to Paris and presenting them with visual evidence of his mastery, Guido communicated his grasp of the art of medicine to his royal patrons.

Islamic Anatomy and European Responses

Despite Guido's exhortations of the value of illustration to anatomical understanding, he was the last European surgeon until the sixteenth century to ensure his anatomical text would be accompanied by images. He was not, however, the last physician of the global Middle Ages to include anatomical images in a manual. The most popular illustrated anatomical treatise in the Middle East was authored by Mansūr ibn Muḥammad ibn Amād ibn Yūsuf ibn Ilyās (*fl.* 1380–1420), physician to the governor of Fars in Timurid Persia, and shares interesting ties with Latin contemporaries.[11]

Written in 1386 in Shiraz, some copies of Mansūr's *Tashrīḥ-i badan-i insān* (Anatomy of the Human Body), more commonly known as *Tashrīḥ-i Mansūr-i* (Mansūr's Anatomy), include six full-body anatomical illustrations that bear a striking resemblance to the squatting Five-Figure Series, each representing the veins, arteries, bones, nerves and muscles, as well as the notable addition of a female figure. They are the earliest full-body anatomical figures made in the Islamic world. As previously discussed, there was no religious ban on representing the body in medieval Islamic medical works; many included sections on anatomy, some supplemented with small schematic diagrams like the cranial sutures and the eyeball.[12] Like the full body figures, these have interesting connections to European versions: the eleventh-century diagram demonstrating the cross-sections of two eyeballs, the optic nerve and, in between, the nose (see illus. 8), which accompanied Alhazen's *Kitāb al-Manāẓir* (Book of Optics), is markedly similar to and pre-dates the Nine-Figure Series version (see illus. 18, 19).[13] These connections indicate a common late-antique graphic ancestor.

While the extent of Mansūr's role in the formation and inclusion of the figures in his treatise is unclear – his text makes only one reference to an accompanying image – there are about seventy extant copies of the diagrams, some of which circulated independently from *Tashrīḥ-i Mansūr-i* either on their own or appended to a different text, like Avicenna's *Canon*.[14] The earliest known illustrated copy of *Tashrīḥ-i Mansūr-i* was completed in 1488 (Bethesda, Maryland, National Library of Medicine, MS P 18). The text consists of an introduction, descriptions of each of the five figures with an accompanying image and a conclusion that explains the compound systems and how the foetus is formed, which is accompanied by a pregnant female figure with a foetus in her uterus (illus. 48). While the veins (illus. 12) are pictured frontally, the bone (illus. 45) and nerve (illus. 46) figures of *Tashrīḥ-i Mansūr-i* differ from their Western counterparts because they are shown from a dorsal view: the squatted body faces away, spinal cord stretching down the back, head tipped backwards at an extreme angle to face the viewer. The decision to picture these two figures from behind is presumably due to the importance of clearly delineating the spinal cord for both systems, as Henry of Mondeville also attempted to do for the bones. Mansūr's sole reference to accompanying images is found in the nerve description, in which he stipulates that pairs of nerves ought to be differentiated by colour.[15] The NLM MS P 18 nerve figure does just that: multicoloured inks are used to show the feathered nerves, which extend from the spinal cord throughout the rest of the body, including the brain.

Although there is no evidence of a backwards nerve figure in the West, there are three European examples of the backwards bone figure, two of which pre-date the composition of *Tashrīḥ-i Mansūr-i*: in an Occitan manuscript (Basel, Universitäts-bibliothek, MS D II 11; illus. 47) and likely German manuscript (Munich, Bayerische Staatsbibliothek, Clm 13042), both dated to the early fourteenth century. The third was probably made in Italy and is roughly contemporary with *Tashrīḥ-i Mansūr-i* (Vatican City, Biblioteca Apostolica Vaticana, MS Pal. lat. 1110).[16] Since the oldest surviving example of the Islamic figure dates to the second half of the fifteenth century, it is possible the direction of influence went from Europe to the Middle East, rather than the more common reverse.[17] However, the text that

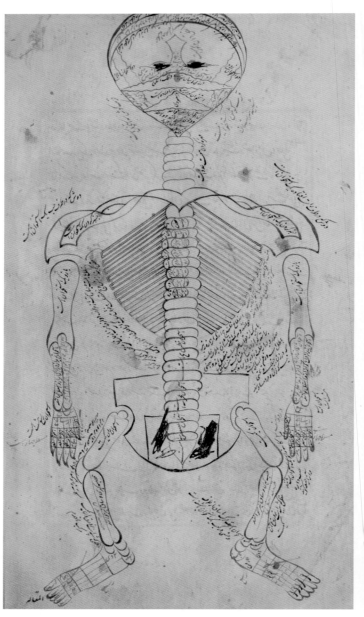

45 Dorsal view of skeleton, from Manṣūr ibn Ilyās, *Tashrīḥ-i Manṣūr-i* (1488).

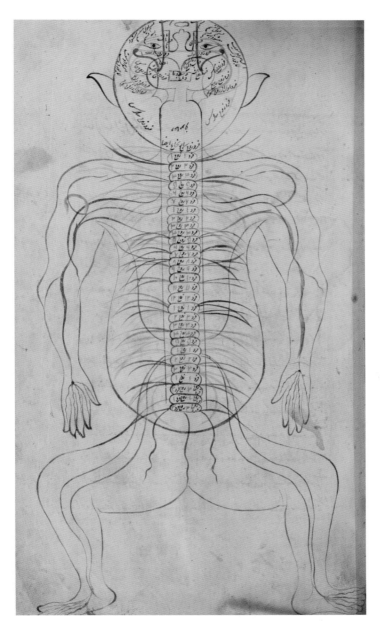

46 Tashrīḥ-i Manṣūr-i Dorsal view of nervous system, from Manṣūr ibn Ilyās, *Tashrīḥ-i Manṣūr-i* (1488).

is written around the bone figures in both the Basel (in Occitan) and Vatican (in Latin) manuscripts, known as *De ossibus corporis* (On the Bones of the Body), is probably Arabic in origin.[18] The only other Western examples of the bone figure were created in very different circumstances. The first, a skeleton found in Clm 13042, is the lone illustration in the entire manuscript, appearing

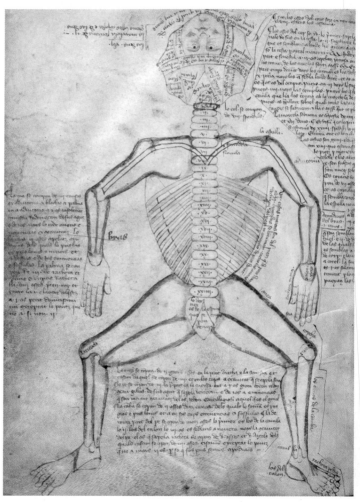

47 Dorsal bone figure, from *Miscellanea medica* [southern France] (c. 1300).

at the end of three scholastic texts that are not strictly medical and so entirely unrelated to the image.[19] The Vatican figure appears with several other unfinished anatomical full-body line drawings, appended as a discrete booklet to the front of a copy of Averroes's *Colliget* (Generalities) of medicine and treatise on a poison antidote.[20] Despite their differences in context, the similarities of the dorsal skeleton in all three Western versions, stylistically and textually, is undeniable.[21] There are still many unknowns regarding this particular confluence of East and West and one can only hope that a scholar well-versed in both traditions will turn their attention to the topic.

It is worth exploring the female figure in the Basel manuscript (see illus. 14) in relation to Mansūr's anatomical woman.[22] While all five of the images in the Basel manuscript borrow some stylistic conventions from the Five-Figure Series – most obviously, the squatting position of the four male bodies – they are unusual in several ways. Only the bone figure is a depiction of a recognizable (and labelled) Galenic system. The remaining four are not captioned and the iconography of their interiors is the only clue we have to identify what specific system – if any – they are meant to represent. The Basel figures are more fluid, displaying different combinations of anatomy within the body over specific functions. Most notably, the female anatomical figure is likely the earliest extant diagram of the internal anatomy of a woman's full body (the only comparable image is the slightly earlier dissected woman in the Ashmole 399 narrative cycle; see illus. 37). The artist has chosen to draw a woman of distinct humanity, with a solemn expression and a respectable red net covering her hair. Her arms are stretched straight out to the sides and red veins run down her neck, arms and torso. She also contains within her outlines what is perhaps the first depiction of the seven-celled uterus (compare it, for instance, to Guido's later version; see illus. 32). Pictured within her torso with the womb are her

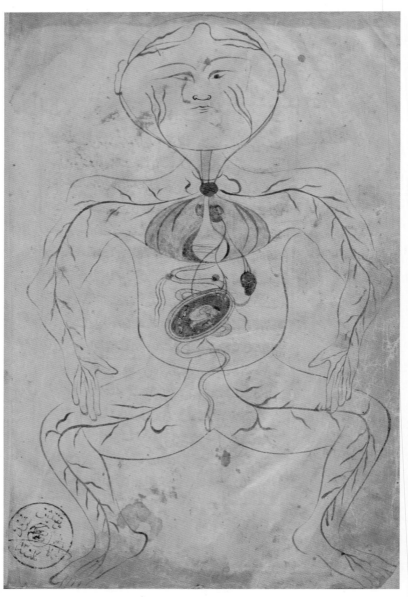

48 Pregnant anatomical woman, from Manṣūr ibn Ilyās, *Tashrīḥ-i Manṣūr-i* (1488).

liver and bladder, connected by veins, all organs thought to play a role in reproduction.

These representations of the seven-celled uterus, as seen in the Basel figure and Guido of Vigevano's, illustrate the longevity of the theory. Mansūr's female figure (illus. 48) more generally resembles the fifteenth-century Disease Woman discussed in Chapter Two (see illus. 30), but does not attempt to label and describe each part in such compartmentalized detail. Rather, Mansūr's female anatomy functions in the same manner as the male vein and artery figures, in which the womb is understood in relation to the movement of the blood throughout the body, an unremarkable and necessary anatomical aspect. In the Basel manuscript, the differences of the female form are highlighted by its placement in opposition to a male figure on the right side of the same opening. He sports a full beard, traditionally associated with masculinity and virility, and his external genitalia is clearly delineated. The juxtaposition of these two images reinforces the role of each sex in reproduction: the woman, her hair conservatively covered, positioned on the weak female left and marked by her uterus, versus the boldly squatting bearded man on the male right, genitalia on proud display.[23]

* * *

The brevity of this chapter on medieval practitioners with illustrated anatomical manuals indicates the uniqueness of Guido of Vigevano and Mansūr ibn Ilyas and their predecessor Henry of Mondeville, as well as the general lack of anatomical illustrations in the fourteenth and fifteenth centuries. This would gradually change in the second half of the fifteenth century as the practice of human dissection spread along with the growth of print as a medium. But after Guido in the mid-fourteenth century, innovation in medieval anatomical imagery was somewhat static. Illustration increasingly became the remit of professional artists, and the establishment of Mondino dei Liuzzi's text as the basis of anatomical teaching left little room for new imagery devised by surgeons themselves, or for the copying of older imagery created by surgeons like Henry and Guido. The notable exception to this is Mansūr's anatomical images, which were reproduced in great numbers in Middle Eastern medical manuals for centuries.

Instead of creating new images or recycling older ones, Western illuminated surgical texts after Guido were mostly commissioned by wealthy patrons and adorned with anatomical images that reflected popular contemporary illustrative tropes. It would not be until the very end of the fifteenth century that new anatomical images were created for epistemic purposes, and several decades after that before another educated surgeon would create his own images to illustrate his anatomical writings.

PART III

ANATOMY AND ARTISTS

Decorating the Text: Professional Artists and the Anatomical Page

I n the absence of the notable rarity of a surgeon like Guido of Vigevano designing anatomical images himself, the task of devising imagery for anatomical texts most often fell to professional workshop artists in the later Middle Ages. It bears repeating that the vast majority of medical texts were unillustrated, and those that were mostly did not contain anatomical images. But in the few surviving examples of professionally illuminated anatomical treatises from the twelfth to the fifteenth centuries, we see the formation of a language of anatomy similar to that found in the liturgical, theological and vernacular manuscripts being creating for an increasingly book-hungry populace in urban areas. Professional illuminators enriched and clarified these texts for wealthy clientele with memorable and colourful graphic divisions, like decorative capital letters (known as historiated initials) and small scenes (miniatures), to signify the start of different chapters and sections.[1] To create relevant, elegant iconography, these artists – almost certainly unfamiliar with the stiff, squatting bodies and abstracted organ diagrams of the Nine-Figure Series, or other images associated with the scholastic surgery tradition – turned to popular contemporary illumination styles to make what I will call 'courtly anatomy': sprightly dissected figures and organs painted against gilded, patterned backgrounds (see illus. 7). We have seen similar figures in the richly illuminated copy of Henry of Mondeville's

surgical manuscript (BnF MS fr. 2030; see illus. 35), although
Henry's role in the creation of these images was the exception
rather than the rule. The dissected figures produced by professional artists do not betray any specific knowledge of the interior,
with a few notable exceptions, like the extraordinarily detailed
images adorning the centre of a fifteenth-century surgical roll
(see illus. 54–7).

The dominance of professional workshops producing and
illustrating texts began in the late twelfth and early thirteenth
centuries. These workshops cohered most notably in Paris, where
the rapid expansion of the University of Paris, coupled with
patronage by French royalty, nobility and religious houses of
the surrounding region, meant that ateliers able to support the
growing demand sprang up around the capital.[2] Although the
University of Paris was most well-known for its theological
faculty, medicine was firmly established there by the early thirteenth century.[3] The types of medical manuscripts professional
artisans were called upon to illustrate were encyclopaedias like
the *De proprietatibus rerum* (On the Properties of Things) by
Bartholomew the Englishman (*fl.* 1220s–70), which was popular
among wealthy elites who were not studying medicine, or lengthy
textbooks such as the late twelfth-century Latin translation of
Avicenna's *Canon* by Gerard of Cremona (c. 1114–1187), consulted by students, physician professors and practitioners. The
images were most often drawn in historiated initials but were
also sometimes included in larger standalone miniatures at the
start of different sections of the text, and, in one memorable
instance, within marginal decoration.

Before proceeding, a caveat: most students would not have
been able to afford the types of illuminated books under discussion here. They would have purchased the texts required by their
curriculum in the form of unadorned booklets (*libelli*), the production of which was closely monitored by the universities to

ensure professional workshops were producing and selling the correct treatises.[4] Furthermore, many students and professors were members of the mendicant orders, unenclosed monks sworn to divest themselves of all worldly goods to spend their time as itinerant preachers, integrating the Church more fully into the everyday lives of those who lived in urban communities.[5] Although their main objective was evangelizing, allowances were made for the friars of both major and minor orders, as well as lay clergy – diocesan priests who were not members of a religious order – to study and teach medicine in universities.[6] However, mendicant medical scholars generally steered clear of surgery and dissection (as the Church forbade those in higher orders especially from spilling any blood[7]) and were also technically discouraged from possessing expensive items like the illuminated books explored here, although there is plenty of evidence to the contrary.

In this chapter, we will consider the different ways in which professional illuminators, with no input (of which we are aware) from surgeons or anatomists, created memorable and entertaining illustrative anatomical images for wealthy patrons. Although these workshop artists most likely did not have any formal education in anatomy, the visual vocabulary they developed would come to define the form and function of anatomical images for centuries, until their fifteenth- and sixteenth-century artistic descendants began to study anatomy themselves.

Encyclopaedic Anatomy

Aside from the new anatomical treatises being written by the rational surgeons around Bologna in the twelfth and thirteenth centuries, there was not much anatomical content in early medical curricula. The most important was the primarily Galenic ideas in the *Pantegni*, augmented by the translation into Latin of Avicenna's *Canon* in the late twelfth century, which would become a foundational medical text by the middle of the thirteenth.[8] The *Canon* featured five books covering everything from descriptions of the humours, elements and temperaments to medical substances, compound remedies and diagnosis and treatment of diseases.[9] Although anatomy was not given its own book or even section within a book, but rather is scattered mostly in Books One and Three, Avicenna's summaries of the form and function of the 'members' were central to university medical education. Galenic and Aristotelian ideas about the body were also incorporated into other popular works created around the universities. The desire to keep up with the latest writings that were coming into Latin Europe for the first time in the twelfth and thirteenth centuries led to the production of exhaustive encyclopaedias of general knowledge and other new works that included human anatomy. The medical sections in these encyclopaedias conformed to the Islamic tradition of condensing medical writings into a single, abridged compendium of reference material *a capite ad calcem* (literally, 'from head to heel'), a format transported to Europe from the Middle East beginning in the eleventh century.[10] New Latin encyclopaedias of general knowledge were mostly created by those studying and teaching within the new university systems, including two notable examples of friars – one Franciscan, one Dominican – producing works that included anatomical sections. The earlier is an encyclopaedia of general knowledge, Bartholomew's *De proprietatibus rerum*, and the second is Albert the Great's (d. 1280) *De animalibus* (On Animals).

Bartholomew produced *De proprietatibus rerum* in several stages during the 1220s and 1230s while he studied and taught at the universities of Paris and Saxony.[11] His encyclopaedia became very popular soon after completion; there are more than two hundred manuscript copies extant in Latin and European vernacular languages, a stunning number attesting to the medieval appetite for wide-ranging knowledge. Bartholomew divided his work into nineteen chapters dedicated to the natural 'things', which ranged from the planets and stars to the human body, animals and minerals, the elements and the nature of God. Three books deal with anatomy: Five (on the parts of the body), Six (on the simple members, that is, bones, veins and hair) and Seven ('Categories of Men and Women', 'Non-Natural' things, and diseases and cures of the body). Bartholomew assiduously noted his sources in the margins where applicable; his most oft-cited medical authorities include Hippocrates, Aristotle, Galen, Avicenna and Constantine the African. Book Five is the most anatomical, beginning with the head and ending, of course, with an image and description of the heel.

None of the extant copies of De proprietatibus rerum include substantial illumination throughout the anatomical parts of the text save for two: one manuscript made in Italy in the first decade of the fourteenth century (London, British Library, Add. MS 8785) and a French manuscript made in the fifteenth century (Paris, Bibliothèque nationale de France, MS fr. 22532).[12] While MS fr. 22532 features clothed, full-body figures to illustrate the organ chapters, Add. MS 8785 is the only known manuscript in the De proprietatibus rerum tradition to include images of small, segmented organs and body parts (illus. 49–51). It was made between 1299 and 1309 at the behest of a councillor of the northern Italian city of Mantua, Vivaldo Belcalzer (fl. 1270s–1309), as a gift to Mantua's signore or ruler, Guido Bonacolsi (d. 1309). The manuscript has the distinction of being both one of the earliest illuminated copies of De proprietatibus rerum and one of the first renderings of the popular encyclopaedia in the vernacular. Translated only seventy or so years after the original was written, Add. MS 8785 attests that the encyclopaedia was already popular enough to have been a desirable acquisition for those who preferred to read in their native tongue over Latin.

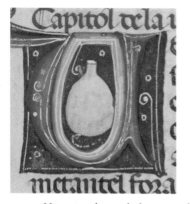 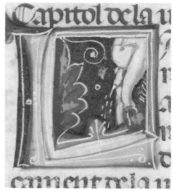

49, 50 Historiated initials featuring the bladder (left) and urinating (right), from Bartholomew the Englishman, *De proprietatibus rerum* (c. 1300–1309).

Nearly all of the illumination in Add. MS 8785 is found in historiated initials. The manuscript is filled with hundreds of them, remarkably uniform and decorating nearly every folio of the manuscript. In the anatomical section, the artist(s) chose to fill each small, bright blue initial background with the organ discussed in that chapter, including the kidneys, liver, stomach, heart, lungs, spleen and gallbladder, among others. They are reminiscent in their simplified disembodiment of some of the organs on the Cambridge organ leaf (see illus. 5) or in the Henry of Mondeville tradition, but while many of those are squeezed together – the Cambridge leaf features eleven – or sketched into marginal spaces, the Add. MS 8785 images are simple, organized and neatly encased within the interior of the initials. In many cases, the Add. MS 8785 organs are so non-specific (especially evident when comparing the bladder (illus. 49) and the womb (illus. 51), which appear to be exactly the same) that they would be unidentifiable without the text and captions describing each image. They were meant to decorate and signpost parts of the text and help the reader to remember what they read, but do not betray any detailed knowledge of human anatomy. Instead, they tap into a general

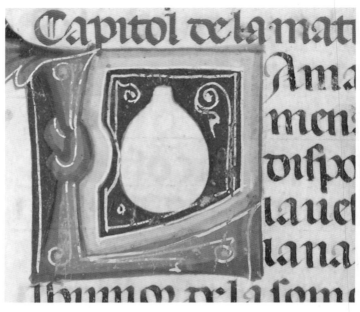

51 Historiated initial featuring the womb, from Bartholomew the
Englishman, *De proprietatibus rerum* (c. 1300–1309).

communal understanding of the forms of the organs of the body
that most readers would be able to recognize. Although unrelated
to surgeons or surgical texts, the Add. MS 8785 organs represent
the type of knowledge on display in the encyclopaedic format,
broken down into initials. Bartholomew's encyclopaedia allowed
his readers to situate all natural things together, each part making
up the whole of the universe according to God's plan.

A uniquely ornate copy of Albert the Great's *De animalibus*
with anatomical drawings was created sometime between the
1330s and 1360s (Bibliothèque nationale de France, MS lat.
16169).[13] Albert had a considerable hand in the formation of
thirteenth-century scholastic philosophy, and his relatively well-
documented life gives us insight into the activities of mendicant
scholars, particularly the travel required for intellectual pursuits
and in service to their order. He was born into a wealthy family

in Bavaria around the year 1200 and studied at the University of Padua. He decided to join the Dominican order in 1223 and went to Cologne to train to be a member, where he also studied theology. After circulating through several schools in Germany, he received his theology degree at the University of Paris in 1245 and commenced teaching again. It was in this period that he attracted his most famous student, Thomas Aquinas, and together they studied new translations of Aristotelian philosophy, attempting to understand and apply Aristotle's writings to contemporary theological issues. While writing extensively, Albert also travelled around the Continent, primarily in Germany, to perform various ecclesiastical duties on behalf of the Dominicans. In addition to writing commentaries on Aristotle's works, Albert authored many of his own. *De animalibus* represented the final level in Albert's divisions of the natural world, which began with the heavens and

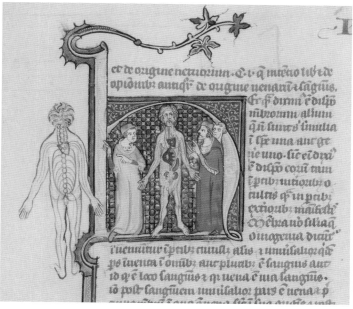

52 Historiated initial featuring frontal and dorsal dissected bodies with academics, from Albert the Great, *De animalibus* (1330–60).

included the earth, minerals and vegetables, and is based on Aristotle's works as well as those of Thomas of Cantimpré (1201–1272).[14] *De animalibus* encompassed more than just a discussion of beasts; it included human anatomy, medicine, reproduction and embryology.

The incorporation of anatomy in the professional decorative programme of MS lat. 16169 is unique in form as well as in terms of the *De animalibus* tradition; it is one of the only copies to include images in the human anatomy and embryology sections, and makes use of the margins as well as historiated initials. In addition to situating a detailed anatomical figure within a historiated initial (illus. 52), the artist(s) drew a headless dissected figure and cluster of organs in the lower margin (illus. 53) instead of the usual animated flora and fauna. The central figure in the margin is an enlarged, opened corpse, flanked by two groups of three capped medical students who gaze up at it, gesturing, as though witnessing a dissection. The faint outline of the cadaver's skin can be seen surrounding the organs. The figure demonstrates, from the top, the throat travelling down to the organs of the thorax and abdomen: the heart surrounded by the lungs; the intestinal coil; five-lobed liver with the blue oval gallbladder, wrapped over the stomach; the oblong spleen; and below, on

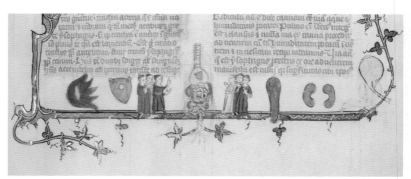

53 Marginalia featuring organs, academics and a dissected torso, from Albert the Great, *De animalibus* (1330–60).

either side of the intestines, the two kidneys. On either side of the figure are enlarged views of several organs: from left, the liver and gallbladder, heart, spleen and pair of kidneys.

The singular arrangement of imagery in this manuscript demonstrates the creativity and playfulness of professional illuminators. Produced in Paris, undoubtedly at considerable cost, it is possible to imagine a successful medical man associated with the university commissioning this stunning copy of Albert's text for his personal use.

Courtly Anatomy

Aside from creating models and figures, Henry of Mondeville also potentially worked with a professional workshop in Paris to produce the decorated 1314 copy of his treatise (BnF MS fr. 2030; see illus. 35). Before Henry, there are only a few examples of Parisian courtly anatomy illustration. The most notable has been attributed to a specific workshop: the Johannes Grusch atelier.[15] The Grusch atelier was active from approximately 1235–70 and responsible for decorating several medical books.[16] The first is a copy of popular mid-thirteenth-century medical texts (Avignon, Bibliothèque municipale, MS 1019), including Gerard of Cremona's translation of Rhazes's *Almansor*, and features thirteen illuminated initials depicting a 'friar physician' (*frater medicus*) performing the duties of a physician professor, analysing urines, instructing students and treating patients.[17] The second manuscript contains the *Articella* (Philadelphia, University of Pennsylvania, Rare Book and Manuscript Library, MS LJS 24) and the illuminations depict another tonsured practitioner, this one attired in the black-and-white robes of the Dominican order.[18] This appears to be the only Dominican-specific illustrated medical treatise of the period, and perhaps the earliest instance of any illustration accompanying the *Articella*.[19] However, these representations do not include images of the friars with dissected bodies, most likely because of the prohibition of friars to shed blood, but may also reflect the rarity of cadaveric dissection in Paris before the end of the fifteenth century.[20]

The Grusch atelier's foray into courtly anatomy is found in a copy of Avicenna's *Canon* created in approximately 1260 (Besançon, Bibliothèque municipale, MS 457).[21] The Besançon manuscript contains a similarly unified, highly decorated image programme like that of the Avignon and Philadelphia manuscripts. In the sections on anatomy, a partially dissected but evidently living body is presented against geometric backgrounds, framed by Gothic architectural elements and enhanced with extensive use of gold leaf (see illus. 7). The dissected bodies are supported by an attendant and strike a variety of poses, while a physician – most likely meant to be Avicenna himself, capped and richly gowned in blue robes and red robes in two separate miniatures – gestures at them. The energetic positioning of the figures evokes a narrative feel, as if illustrating the physician's encounter with a specific patient, rather than an imagined scene. The imagery recalls the Henry of Mondeville figures in BnF MS fr. 2030, but with a more structured division of labour reflecting the idea that a dissection was performed by an uneducated barber-surgeon and presided over by the physician-professor.

There is only one fourteenth-century Italian example (to my knowledge) containing this type of courtly anatomical imagery: a luxurious two-volume set of Avicenna's *Canon* (Vatican City, Biblioteca Apostolica Vaticana, MSS Urb. lat. 240 and 241).[22] Book One (Urb. lat. 241) describes the anatomy of the parts of the body, and each chapter heading includes a colourful historiated initial featuring either a patient gesturing to the relevant part under discussion. Most remarkably, some initials depict a seated physician (again, likely meant to be Avicenna) holding an organ while explaining it to a student or disciple, a unique combination of the courtly anatomy scenes found in Parisian illumination with the organ initials of the Italian Add. MS 8785.

Anatomy Outside the Hierarchy of the Page

The previous examples demonstrate the ways in which anatomical imagery fit into the regulated framework of the scholastic page: within initials or as marginal images, specific decoration that conformed to expectations for manuscript illumination. But there are a few examples of professional productions of anatomical images that eschewed these constraints.

The first we will explore is the remarkable 5-metre-long (16 ft) fifteenth-century Stockholm Roll (National Library of Sweden, MS X 188).[23] The roll features four full-body anatomical images in the central margin between two columns of text and four on the back of the roll (illus. 54–7). The images are only vaguely related to the text of the scroll – the popular *De arte phisicali et de cirurgia* (On the Art of Medicine and Surgery) of John of Arderne (1307/8–d. in or after 1377) and *Practica* of fistula-in-ano – and seem instead to function as striking, provocative decoration for a wealthy patron. It was clearly an expensive commission, perhaps meant for the English princess Philippa, who was married to Eric of Pomerania, king of Norway and Sweden.[24]

The Stockholm Roll iconography is a mixture of some (rather titillating) drawings of the removal of anal fistulas, which are reminiscent of Arderne's but not exactly those associated with his treatise, and animated images of well-heeled patients receiving medical care as well as the large and vibrant anatomical figures. The roll also includes fifteen drawings of foetuses in the womb associated with Muscio (as in illus. 9). Created in London circa 1425–35, the roll is comprised of twelve pieces of parchment sewn together. The majority of the richly painted figures

– numbering nearly one hundred – are smaller and decorate the outer margins and spaces between the larger anatomical figures, which are situated in the central margin, flanked by the two columns of text. The artist used both sides of the scroll for frontal and dorsal views of the four figures: a vein man, a skeleton (illus. 54–5), a nerve figure (although this is unclear) and the bisected man (illus. 56–7). The last is the most striking: a man pulling his ribcage apart to demonstrate his interior. His face has been sliced in half, blood dribbling from the divide. He

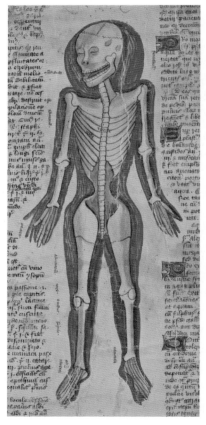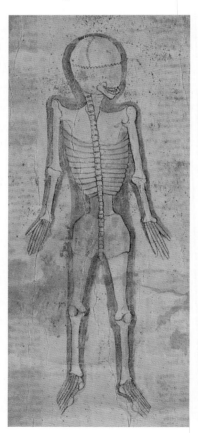

54, 55 Skeleton (left: front of scroll; right: dorse of scroll), from John Arderne, *De arte phisicali et de chirurgia* (c. 1425–35).

displays his heart and lungs, liver and green gallbladder, pink stomach, brown spleen and blue, red and yellow coils of his intestines. Even his penis has been bisected. The view painted directly behind him on the dorse of the roll presents a different perspective, with kidneys visible and black swirls of intestines dominating the abdomen. Blood drips down his buttocks and thighs.

John of Arderne was the most famous English surgeon of the Middle Ages. Although he was a considerably learned practitioner, quoting extensively from popular surgical treatises in his works, he does not appear to have ever been enrolled in a university. He describes treating noblemen for their anal fistula, detailing the sums he was able to command, and the number of copies that survive of his works, illustrated and unillustrated, is a testament to his renown not only during his lifetime, but posthumously.[25] The *Practica* is notable as an illustrated treatise and Arderne makes frequent references to the accompanying images in his text, indicating he had a first-hand role in creating them.[26] But unlike many of his southern European predecessors and contemporaries – notably, Mondino dei Liuzzi and Guy of Chauliac – Arderne did not include an account of anatomy in his surgical manual.[27] It is curious, then, that the Stockholm Roll features the four anatomical figures as the largest and most striking of all the illustrations. The unique presence of back views of the four figures (and one fistula-in-ano) on the dorse of the scroll, in the same place as the frontal views, further underlines their significance. Why include anatomical images on an expensive scroll when they were unrelated to the text?

Although it is tempting to force a link between these images and those we have discussed, they seem instead to be unique outliers to other learned anatomical traditions while at the same time exhibiting a higher level of anatomical detail (exaggerated though it may be) than the majority of those produced by other

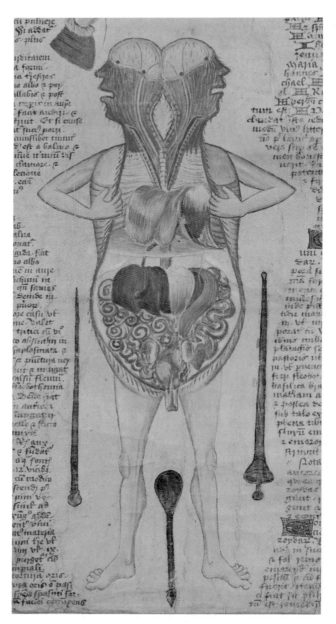

56, 57 Bisected man (above: front of scroll; opposite: dorse of scroll), from John Arderne, *De arte phisicali et de chirurgia* (c. 1425–35).

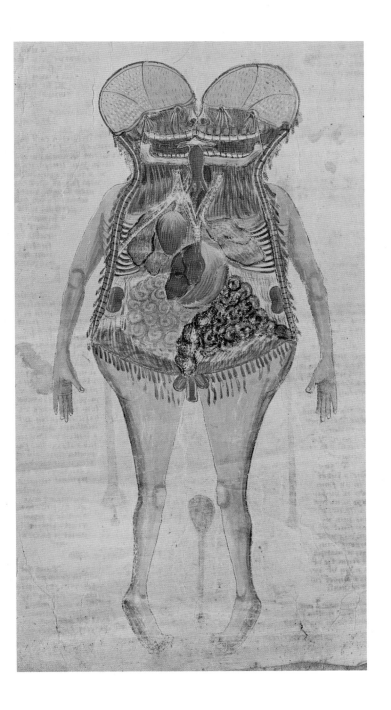

professional artists. The closest potential ancestors of the
Stockholm images within the bounds of learned anatomy are
the frontal and dorsal views of the body attached to Henry of
Mondeville's anatomical treatise (see illus. 35, 39, 40); but any
similarities between those small, simplified drawings in a codex
with these large and vibrant scroll figures are minor. Instead, the
Stockholm images exhibit tropes of contemporary images not
associated with medical treatises, featuring the sort of macabre
body humour popular in later medieval illumination: the smiling
memento mori skeletons associated with the Dance of Death,
for instance (such as the frescoes created for an Estonian church
at the end of the fifteenth century; illus. 58). Arderne's popularity
hinged on his appeal to both 'high' and 'low' practitioners, to
scholastic and everyday surgical traditions. He chose to write his
text in Latin and refer to the learned surgical tradition, while
at the same time peppering his text with his own 'chatty' narra-
tives of patients and treatments he had experienced at first hand,
and useful yet inevitably bawdy images of rear ends. Arderne's
figures clearly demonstrate the practical points of treating anal
fistula, while, at the same time, acting as ludic marginalia might
within religious manuscripts: titillating and memorable for a non-
medical viewer.[28] Likewise, the grinning skeleton and aggrieved
bisected man on the Stockholm Roll keep the viewer's focus on
the function and make-up of the body while also ensuring a memorable encounter with human anatomy. One can imagine the
scroll as something consulted by a physician, enjoyed as an art
object by a patron, or perhaps even both.

Several of the Stockholm images have stylistic connections
to a set of six frontal and dorsal figures added to the end of a
compilation of anatomical texts in Latin and English (London,
Wellcome Library, MS 290).[29] The texts date to the mid-fifteenth
century,[30] while the images are almost certainly later; the two
final figures – the pregnant Disease Woman (see illus. 72) and

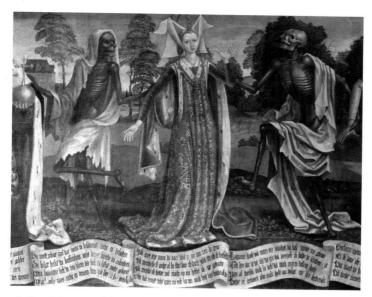

58 Detail from workshop of Bernt Notke, *Dance of Death*, late 15th century, oil and tempera on canvas.

the Wound Man – were copied from the printed medical text *Fasciculus medicinae*, which first appeared in 1491.[31] The skeleton (illus. 59, 60), with frontal and dorsal views together in the same opening, is particularly reminiscent of the Stockholm Roll images, surrounded by a black outline, red in the Stockholm skeletons. As both were likely created by professional artists in London, they speak to a persistent graphic technique and were even perhaps made within the same scriptorium, a few decades apart.

Artist-Anatomist

After about the mid-fifteenth century, learned anatomical images began to move from the hands of workshop illuminators into those of people who worked in different media. The relationship

overleaf: 59, 60 Frontal and dorsal skeletons, from *Miscellanea medica* [England] (late 15th century).

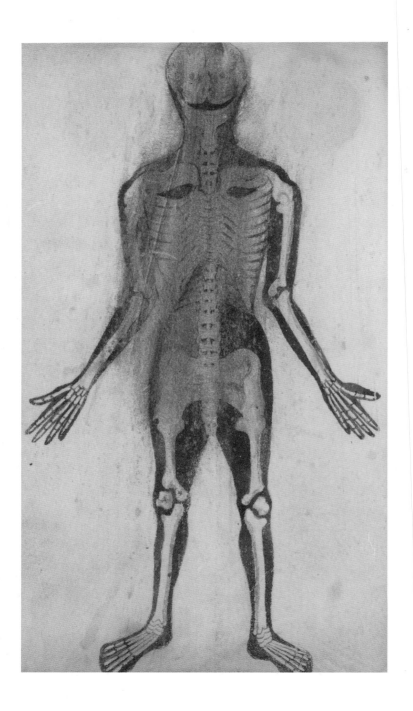

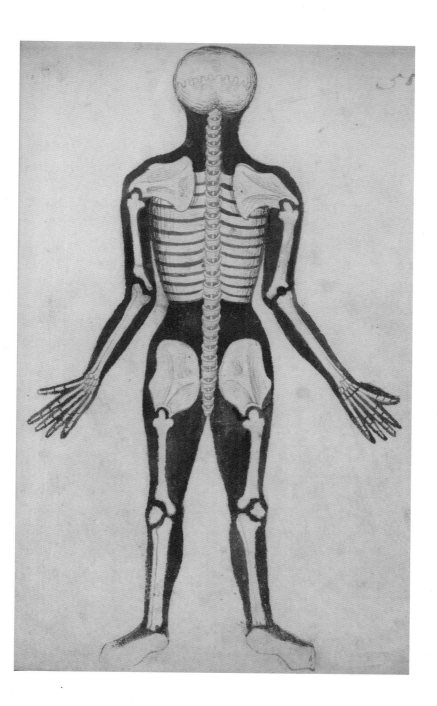

between professional artists and anatomists, exemplified by Henry of Mondeville and Guido of Vigevano in the fourteenth century, evolved into collaborations instigated by artists rather than anatomists in the later fifteenth century, as accurately depicting human anatomy became increasingly important to fresco and panel painters and sculptors. This in turn prompted some university anatomists to re-evaluate both the importance of images in their written works as well as the form of the images themselves: the imagined, technical or abstract diagram was slowly supplanted by realistic depictions of the interior of the body, idealized but mirroring reality. These images, along with the collaboration between anatomist and artist, would become as important as the anatomical texts themselves. Overall, this transformation of aesthetic priorities has been described as a shift from memorial – geared towards memorization, or relying on and playing to memory – to documentary culture.[32]

The discussion of art and anatomy in the fifteenth and six-teenth centuries is an enormous subject on which much has already been written. In keeping with this book's focus on text-based anatomical images, the remainder of this chapter will be dedicated to examples of professional late medieval artists who chose to dissect corpses and engage with anatomical texts in order to more realistically depict the body, as well as learned anatomists who trained as artists and used their skills to illustrate their works.

In his *Commentaries* (c. 1447), the influential Florentine artist Lorenzo Ghiberti (1378–1455) argued that it was necessary for an artist 'to have seen the works [of Hippocrates and Avicenna and Galen] and to have seen a dissection [*notomia*], to know the number of all the bones there are in the human body, to know the muscles in it, to know all the nerves and all the ligaments that are in the male figure'.[33] Ghiberti's statement indicates several things: first, that dissection was accessible enough in mid-fifteenth-century Italy as to be something that non-medical students could witness; second, an artist did not need to be a physician, but to achieve true success, one had to understand what lay beneath the skin; and third, by mentioning the works of Hippocrates, Avicenna and Galen, Ghiberti suggests that although one might witness a human dissection, the elite artist understood that such a demonstration must be supplemented by reading the descriptions of human anatomy recorded by the medical authorities canonized in the field over the course of the Middle Ages.

Fifteenth-century Italian paintings and sculptures of the human body reflect both the persistence of the memorial purpose of images, particularly portraiture, as well as the growing importance of mimetic or naturalistic representation, broadly defined as works that attempt to depict reality through close attention to proportion, perspective and detail.[34] During this period in western Europe, the status of the professional artist increased to the extent that painters went from being mostly anonymous workshop collaborators to recognized individuals who gained fame for their skills, and who were judged primarily on their ability to realistically depict an idealized version of the human form. An example frequently pointed to as a turning point in artistic representation of human anatomy is the fresco of the *Holy Trinity* in Santa Maria Novella in Florence (*c.* 1427; illus. 61) by the Florentine artist Masaccio (1401–1428).[35] Below the depiction of Christ on the Cross lies a skeleton upon a tomb, above which are the words: 'I once was what you are and what I am you also will be' (*Io fui gia quell che voi siete e quell ch'io sono voi ancor sarete*). The skeleton does not resemble contemporary imagery associated with learned anatomy; rather, it indicates both study by Masaccio of parts of a human skeleton as well as a continued reliance on presenting a recognizable, perfected *idea* of a skeleton.[36]

Towards the turn of the sixteenth century, there is some evidence of Italian artists collaborating with surgeons and anatomists

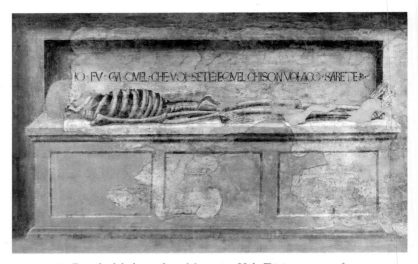

61 Detail of skeleton from Masaccio, *Holy Trinity*, c. 1427, fresco, Santa Maria Novella, Florence.

to view (and, in some cases, participate in) human dissections. Although it is certainly possible that earlier artists did so as well, especially those based around universities where dissections were occurring with relative frequency, we do not have extensive evidence of a direct relationship between human dissections and professional artists until Leonardo da Vinci.[37] Leonardo is considered today to be the archetypal Renaissance genius, a polymath who devoted himself to a wide variety of intellectual and artistic pursuits, and his fame now and during his own lifetime means his life and activities are relatively well-documented. He approached the study of human anatomy differently than his contemporaries because he was interested in not only capturing the musculature for artistic purposes, but in understanding physiology by conducting his own experiments on the human body.[38] He is said to have performed autopsies in the hospital of Santa Maria Nuova between approximately 1505 and 1510. He also evidently worked with a professor of anatomy at the University of Padua, Marcantonio della Torre, to dissect bodies, from which his most detailed anatomical studies emerged. His drawings betray an interest in almost all aspects of the interior of the human body, and he sketched separate parts over and over again, perfecting his mastery of muscles and ligaments and the situation of organs. But Leonardo's images were not simply direct representations of dissected bodies. They reveal his artistic preoccupations with symmetry and form, and often he omitted elements that might hide aspects of the part he wished to depict.[39] This can be seen in his drawings of the uterus, which do not depict the stomach and intestines (see illus. 13). These works, made privately, were unknown to the public until they were published more than a century later; they were for his own personal use and understanding.

Although Leonardo worked within the academic realm, other well-known Italian artists were not as interested in understanding physiology and studied anatomy to advance their artistic skills. Michelangelo (1475–1564) allegedly attended private dissections, according to an account by one of his students, but there is no evidence he explored anatomy on an academic level, while Raphael (1483–1520) studied and worked from skeletons that were hung by hooks to accurately depict bone structure, upon which he layered muscle and skin.[40]

Jacopo Berengario of Carpi (c. 1460–c. 1530), a Modenese surgeon who became the chair of surgery at the University of Bologna, published two of the most famous illustrated anatomical treatises before Vesalius.[41] He was also the next surgeon after Guido of Vigevano to create new anatomical images for his surgical manual. His *Isagogae breves* (Short Introduction to Anatomy), published in 1522 and again in 1523, included 21 woodcuts.[42] Berengario trained as a printmaker before studying medicine, and so when it came time for him to compose his own treatise, he chose to show off his artistic skills and his familiarity with human anatomy. Despite being visually striking, the anatomical information demonstrated by many of his figures is almost

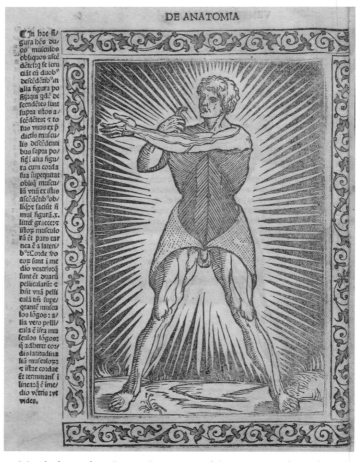

62 Muscle figure, from Jacopo Berengario of Carpi, *Isagogae brevis* (1523).

non-existent, as seen in images like the muscle man écorché (illus. 62), an idealized, heroic figure surrounded by a corona, arms and legs rippling with muscles, a living flayed body. The anatomy conveyed by this figure is comparable to the Five-Figure Series muscle man (see illus. 20) of some three hundred years before, in which the muscles are a bright red, symmetrical design on the squatting body. Explanatory captions, which would have rendered them more intelligible, were not included on the

Ashmole figure. Similarly, the muscles revealed by Berengario's skinned man are little more than a pattern of hatch marks. The point of Berengario's images seems to have been to communicate what he called an 'anatomy of the senses', a philosophical take not unlike the monastic conception of anatomical imagery as a tool for meditation rather than an independent source of information.[43] However, Berengario did dispute several aspects of Galenic anatomy, most notably in his refutation of the existence of Galen's *rete mirabile*, the 'glorious web' of veins in the forehead, based on the 'hundreds' of bodies he claimed to have dissected. As an artist-anatomist, Berengario straddled the divide between those who engaged with anatomy for the betterment of their artistic skills and those who worked with anatomists to produce images for medical texts.

The first printed scene claiming to be directly based on a live dissection sums up the complicated relationship between anatomists, printers and artists in the early fifteenth century. Images of single objects or events, known as 'counterfeits' (*contrafacts*), became popular in northern Europe, acting in some ways as photographs do today by providing a snapshot of a particular item or episode on a single leaf of paper that could easily circulate and be widely disseminated.[44] In 1517 a counterfeit broadside printed by Johannes Schott in Strasbourg featured a corpse opened from chin to genitals (see illus. 11). The text accompanying the image describes a dissection performed in Strasbourg by the German physician Wendelin Hock (*fl.* 1513–35), who trained at the University of Bologna and sought to advertise his learning and skills by staging one of the first public dissections in German lands. Hock invited local barbers and surgeons to witness the dissection and presumably hoped the counterfeit would remind those who had attended of his talents and trumpet them to those who had not. Despite the naturalistic touches in the drawing – the shading lends three dimensionality, and the brain views are most likely

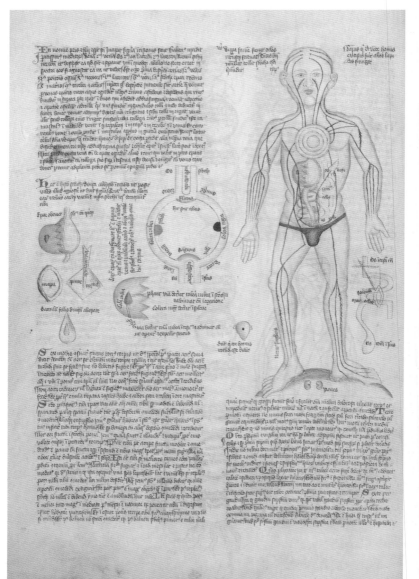

63 Detail of vein figure and internal organs, from the 'Wellcome Apocalypse' (c. 1425).

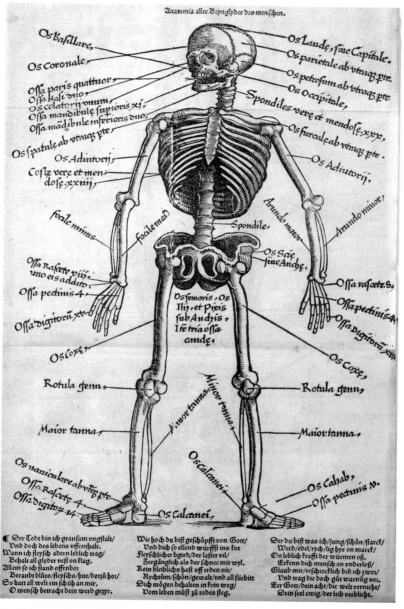

Anatomia aller Beynglyder des menschen.

Os Basillare,
Os Coronale,
Ossa paris quattuor,
Ossa kasi duo,
Os colatorÿ vnum,
Ossa mandibule supioris xj.
Ossa madibule inferioris duo,
Os spatule ab vtraq pte
Os Adiutorÿ,
Coste vere et men-
dose xxiiij,
focile minus
focile maius
Ossa Rasete vij,
uno eis adduo,
Ossa pectinis 4,
Ossa digitorû xv.
Os Cofe,
Rotula genu,
Maior tanna,
Os nauiculare ab vtraq pte
Ossa Rasete 4,
Ossa digitorû 14,
Os Calcanei,

Os Laude, siue Capitale,
Os parietale ab vtraq pte
Os petrosum ab vtraq pte
Os Occipitale,
Spondiles vere et mendose xxxv,
Os furcale ab vtraq pte,
Os Adiutorÿ,
Arundo maior
Arundo minor,
Spondile,
Os Sacie siue Anche,
Ossa rasete S,
Ossa pectinis 4,
Ossa digitorû xv,
Os Coxe,
Rotula genu,
Maior tanna,
Os Cahab,
Ossa pectinis xv.
Os Calcanei,

Os femoris, OS
Ilij, et Pixis
sub Anchis.
I ste tria ossa
caude,

Minor tanna
Minor tanna

64 'Ein contrafacter Todt', woodcut in Hans von Gersdorff,
Feldtbüch der Wundartzney (1528).

based on first-hand observation – the anatomical details reveal their medieval origins. This is especially visible in the sharply pointed, five-lobed liver clutching the stomach in the left side of the torso, which is unmistakably similar to the Wellcome MS 49 imagery from nearly a century before (illus. 63).

This broadside formed a pair with a print of a skeleton (illus. 64), which, we are told by the caption beneath, was based on a skeleton sculpted onto the Saverne tomb of Albrecht, Bishop of Strasbourg from 1478 to 1506, by the artist Nikolaus Hagenauer (d. before 1538).[45] Unfortunately, the tomb sculpture has been lost and so a direct comparison is impossible, but the fact that the caption explicitly links the two – declaring that the skeleton, ironically circulating with the first printed material claiming to be drawn from a live human dissection, was based on a sculpture – reveals that the hundred years between Masaccio's skeleton and Hock's did not see that much of a change in priority for anatomical images. The counterfeit skeleton is an upright, animated view of the bones; a living skeleton, which would remind the surgeons who read the counterfeit, as well as any visitors to Bishop Albrecht's tomb, of the immediacy of death, and the importance of behaving as if one would be standing before St Peter at the gates of heaven imminently. These sixteenth-century artists called upon physical anatomy and spiritual concerns to create images realistic for educational purposes and religious decoration. Indeed, the title at the top of the printed page is 'A Counterfeit Death' ('Ein contrafacter Todt') and the poem below the skeleton reflects upon mortality.

* * *

The juxtaposition of traditionally defined Renaissance artists with medieval ones in this chapter allows us to reconsider the divide between the two, implemented and reinforced by centuries

of scholarship arguing for their stark differences. The factors
that led to the shift from 'two-dimensional' anatomical illustration, in which expressing anatomical function was more
important than form, to 'three-dimensional', in which the physical arrangement of the body's interior was the priority, were
indeed significant. But as has become clear here, I hope, the interest in the accurate portrayal of the body's interior was gradual,
and even those images created purportedly as faithful representations of dissected bodies were still reliant upon unrealistic
viewpoints or graphics to express ideas, the hallmarks of medieval
anatomical figures. This is especially evident in depictions of
skeletons, which remained gruesomely exaggerated in order to
evoke moralistic ideas of the inevitability of death and the use-
lessness of earthly vanity and greed, beliefs that were ever present
in late medieval and early modern imagery and consciousness.

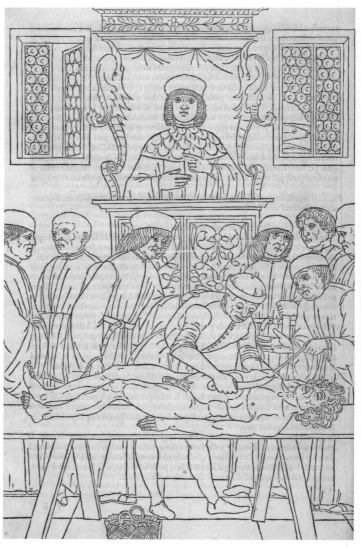

65 Dissection scene, woodcut preceding Mondino dei Liuzzi's *Anathomia* in *Fasciculo de medicina* (1493/4).

SIX

The Anatomy of a Scene: Dissection in Manuscript and Print, c. 1400–1540

The medieval anatomical images discussed so far have mostly used the template of the body as the vehicle for communicating anatomical, physiological or prophylactic information, or presented disembodied but often abstracted views of specific organs and their functions. These figures have largely been anonymous, either inherited from older traditions or devised by unknown workshop artists, and incorporated textual captions to explain their purpose and/or instructions for treatment. The previous chapter's exploration of the diversification of the creators of anatomical images in the late fifteenth and early sixteenth centuries – as anatomical images moved from purely academic contexts into artistic spheres – also occurred among the consumers of anatomical images. Once only available to wealthy, university-educated male viewers, as printing became more affordable, members of the public interested in knowing more about their health collected printed medical texts. The outbreak of plague, beginning with the devastating Black Death pandemic of 1349, saw the profile of physicians rise; they became increasingly important to towns and cities desperate to curb the spread of disease, and to a populace eager to know the best ways to stay healthy and combat infection.[1] Furthermore, physicians prescribed regimens of bloodletting and made dietary and environmental recommendations based on a personalized assessment of someone's unique make-up, computed by considering their zodiac charts, sex and other features unique to each patient.[2] To meet growing demand for medical materials, the earliest printers produced their own versions of popular medical texts, sometimes coupled with a few images at additional expense for the purchaser. The scenes selected for early printed treatises (known as incunabula) are a good indication of the popularity of certain iconographies, but many were also chosen because they were easily reproduced.[3]

In this period of transition, the iconography that became most associated with the field of anatomy was not a view of the interior, labelled with explanations, but rather the act of human dissection itself.[4] Although the details varied from hand to hand, printer to printer and place to place, the basics of the image remained the same: a corpse laid out on a table in the course of being dissected, surrounded by various medical men. The focus was the process of cadaveric dissection as a scholarly enterprise, one that complemented medical study for students. It came to be recognized as a sign of medical competency as the practice gained in popularity in the late fifteenth and early sixteenth centuries.

The standalone diagrams of the Nine-Figure Series and dissected bodies like Henry of Mondeville's did not entirely disappear during this time, as evidenced by the counterfeit broadsheet of the dissected corpse first printed in 1517 (see illus. 11) and subsequently reprinted and reused for years after, which incorporates captions within a dissected cadaver in an effort to add some realism to the format. But the depiction of the act of dissection achieved a level of popularity that transcended the university. By the time the first medical texts were printed in the second half of the fifteenth century, the scene had become the token image associated with anatomical treatises. It took on mythic proportions with the publication of Andreas Vesalius's *Fabrica* (1543), chosen by Vesalius as the image preceding his text (see illus. 41).[5]

In the *Fabrica*'s preface, Vesalius positioned himself as the 'restorer' of anatomy to the glory of antiquity, attacking the dissection techniques of his contemporaries and medieval predecessors, who delegated the act of cutting open the corpse to a lesser surgeon. This traditional method, pictured in the 1493/4 Italian translation of the popular printed *Fasciculus medicinae* (illus. 65), features the lecturer above the dissection, reading from Mondino's anatomical text, while the ostensor with the pointer on the right gestures to the organs and directs the dissector. Vesalius's frontispiece directly attacks this tripartite division of labour, emphasizing his different approach to his readers by memorializing his hands-on technique as the very first part of his treatise. Vesalius remains calm amid a chaotic crush of people clamouring to witness the young anatomist dissect a female corpse, finger raised as he instructs the crowd, the evidence of his knowledge and skill – his knives – on the table next to him.[6]

The intention here is not to frame the *Fabrica* as the culmination of medieval anatomy, as it has so often been designated. But Vesalius's frontispiece is a useful ending point for this discussion because the iconography is a marked contrast to those of his contemporaries and symbolizes the establishment of cadaveric dissection – marginalized in medieval universities for so long – as the most important aspect of medical education. It also recalls Guido of Vigevano's images. Despite his own and some subsequent attempts to paint his achievements as entirely new, Vesalius in fact drew upon decades of precedent in his work and his art when composing his *Fabrica*, the roots of which lie in the thirteenth century.

In this chapter, we will trace the development of the dissection scene in manuscripts and incunabula, exploring what the differences in medium, format, location and context can reveal about changes in anatomical learning and imagery in the late Middle Ages and start of the early modern period. A standalone image of a body being opened first appears in the context of post-mortem examinations some three hundred years before, as explored in Chapter Three, and became associated with the anatomical sections of popular medical and surgical manuscripts in the fourteenth and fifteenth centuries, notably Avicenna's *Canon* and Guy of Chauliac's *Chirurgia magna*. A hallmark of these images is the almost complete absence of recognizable interior anatomy in the corpse's opened cavities; a tangle of intestines was often the extent of what could be gleaned from peering inside. Instead, the focus is on the act itself, rather than the anatomy. We will discover how this scene became canonized as the 'icon' of the field of anatomy, and how Vesalius's frontispiece both drew upon and broke from these visual precedents.

Dissections across Manuscript and Print

One can imagine a wealthy patron's delight on receiving the highly decorated French manuscript edition of Bartholomew the Englishman's *De proprietatibus rerum* (Paris, Bibliothèque nationale de France, MS fr. 218), made in Poitiers in the last quarter of the fifteenth century.[7] The manuscript features easy, flowing script surrounded by glittering foliate borders. The eye is transfixed by the jewel-box scenes painted by skilful professional artists at the start of each of Bartholomew's nineteen books. Would the patron have lingered on the image at the start of Book Five – a corpse laid on a wooden table, being dissected as five men watch and engage in animated discussion (see illus. 6)?

Although this image represents the very highest level of manuscript painting, it was not, in fact, an original composition by an illuminator. Instead, the scribal inscription on this manuscript's final folio declares it to be a copy of a printed edition of the same text, produced in Lyon by 'maistre Jehan Cyber, maistre en l'art d'impression' ('Master Jean Syber, master of the art of printing').⁸ The similarity between the dissection scenes (and indeed all of the images) in MS fr. 218 and Syber's printed version is unmistakable (illus. 66).⁹ Even a cursory comparison of the images reveals a connection, from the overall composition and positions of the figures to their specific gestures and actions. Manuscript and print iconographies in the early days of printing were often in dialogue with each other like this; artists copied manuscript images to carve into woodblocks for printing, and printed images served as models for manuscript artists to paint.¹⁰ In addition, BnF MS fr. 218's colophon adds to our understanding of the relationship between printing workshops. Syber worked in Lyon with Mathieu Hutz, who printed the first French translations, illustrated with woodcuts in 1482.¹¹ While Syber's edition of *Livre des propriétés des choses* is undated, he evidently borrowed the woodblocks from fellow Lyon printer Guillaume Le Roy's edition of 1485/6, who in turn copied Hutz's designs.¹² Although we do not know the identity of the original owner of BnF MS fr. 218,

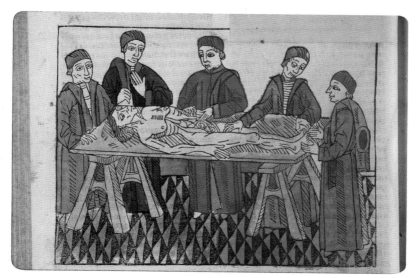

66 Dissection scene, from Bartholomew the Englishman, *Livre des propriétés des choses* (1482).

one possible scenario is that they saw the printed edition of the text and commissioned a workshop to produce a lavish manuscript version. While incunabula were still comparatively expensive works in the 1480s, those that could afford better continued to commission manuscripts as more personalized luxury objects with vibrant and gilded adornment.[13] Indeed, BnF MS fr. 218 must have cost a small fortune, and eventually ended up in the library of a member of the French royal family in the early seventeenth century.

Despite the fact that the dissection image does not reveal much about the body's interior – the opened abdomen in the printed version exposes a knot of intestines, which is reduced to a solid red void in the manuscript – it is still significant as a representation of the way in which a dissection was both imagined by artists and how it actually occurred in educated medical circles. The teacher stands between the two men, probably surgeons, who are physically handling the body. In the manuscript scene, he is older than the others, with long grey hair and whiskers, his ample paunch accented by a wide orange belt. He holds a pointer and instructs the dissectors on how to proceed. They touch the cadaver with familiarity; the man on the far left tenderly cradles the head, and the dissector drawing the knife down the abdomen also grips the left arm. The two men at the end of the table – perhaps students – are engaged in a heated debate. A dog waits hopefully for spills or dropped viscera in the foreground. The printed scene omits some details but is the same compositionally. The inclusion of this scene in both manuscript and print versions of Bartholomew's encyclopaedia whets the viewer's interest for the descriptions of the human body that follow, and encourages the reader to believe – accurately or not – that the author's description was based upon what he had observed during dissection. It is also notable that the scene only appears in printed versions of Bartholomew's work that were made in Lyon; the earliest versions of *De proprietatibus rerum* printed elsewhere were not illustrated.

Manuscript Roots

The general composition of the dissection scene began to take shape as early as the thirteenth century, as explored in Chapter Three with the English Ashmole 399 and the Spanish *Cantigas de Santa María* and their depictions of autopsies. Those miniatures were depictions of private autopsies, not dissections performed for didactic purposes, but the line between the two was continually blurred. Autopsies gained footing as acceptable and useful practices for legal reasons in the thirteenth century; the first recorded public opening of the body (of the criminal Azzolino in 1302) in medieval Europe was as an autopsy. They also became matters of public health, in which professional physicians and other educated medical men were called to perform post-mortem examinations on those suspected of being poisoned by contamination that might affect others. Other types of bodily openings began to be depicted in non-medical manuscript illustration, the most famous being Nero's order that his mother Agrippina to be cut open so he could see his place of origin in her womb, from the popular *Roman de la rose* (for example, the late fifteenth-century scene in the British Library, Harley MS 4425; illus. 67). Many of these images, like that in Harley MS 4425, are gruesome and detailed, in the vein of the Stockholm Roll images.

Aside from the *Cantigas* and Ashmole autopsies, there are few medical manuscript drawings of cadavers being opened, and their identification as either autopsy or dissection is inconclusive. They take place in interior settings, some explicitly private, like a bedchamber, others less certain. They depict simultaneously two legitimized and respected practices, both of which formed part of the important work carried out by experienced surgeons and physicians. Instead of a practitioner alone with a corpse, as in Guido's images, these dissection/autopsy scenes include spectators as well, underscoring the importance of the procedure within medical study (for students) and as a practice of general fascination (for the public).

Perhaps the earliest image of the prototypical dissection scene is found in a French manuscript copy of Guy of Chauliac's *Chirurgia magna*, dating to around 1450–75 (BnF, MS fr. 396; illus. 68). Although it is heavily damaged, it shows a partially dissected corpse laid on a table. Four figures surround the cadaver, each with a hand inside the opened chest. Visible through the

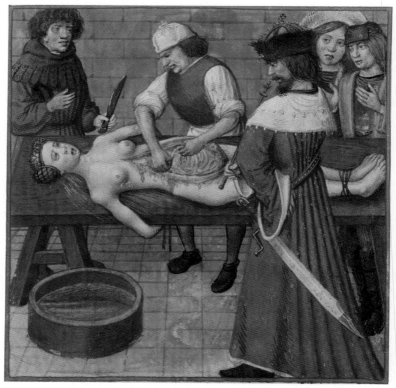

67 'Death of Agrippina', from Jean de Meun, *Roman de la rose* (c. 1490–1500).

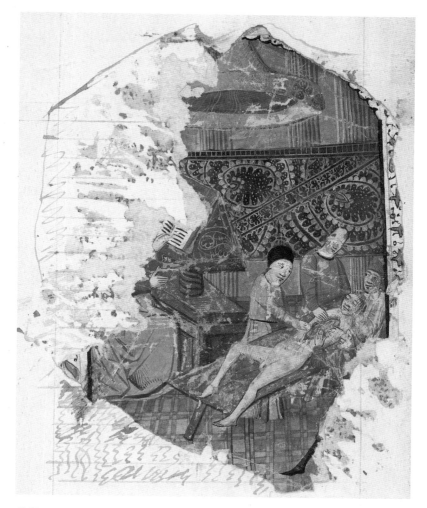

68 Dissection scene, from Guy of Chauliac, *La grande chirurgie* (c. 1450–75).

damage on the left side of the miniature is an enlarged figure seated in a professor's chair (or *cathedra*) before an open book. This aspect– along with the placement of the image within a surgical manual – indicates this is probably meant to depict a scientific human dissection rather than an autopsy, but of course this is not certain.[14] Another example of a similar scene is found in a later French copy of the same text (Montpellier, Bibliothèque universitaire de médecine, MS H 184; illus. 69). Appearing at the start of Book One, the miniature is the width of two columns of text and surrounded by a gilded foliate border. Its style and decoration as well as the types of clothing worn by the figures indicate a French or Flemish origin and a date of circa 1480–1500, but nothing else is known about the manuscript's creation.[15] Some fourteen people crowd the room, those at the back craning their heads to see the action taking place on a wooden table in the foreground, where an enlarged corpse is positioned. The central standing figure – black hair flowing beneath a bright red cap – removes the curling intestines from the corpse's abdomen, while to his right another cuts the cadaver's throat, peeling back a flap of skin. A figure holding a bucket stands in the foreground to catch the organs as they are removed, and beside him is a small bench with various tools for dissection, including a hammer and a large curved blade.

Like BnF MS fr. 396, the Montpellier scene could also depict an autopsy; indeed, it seems more likely in this case that it does.[16] It clearly takes place within the bedchamber of a wealthy person, the upper left side of the miniature occupied by a red bed, accented with gold leaf. Three women are among those present: two of them, garbed in green with their hair covered, stand to the left of the table, and a third appears to be praying next to the bed. A man in blue trimmed with ermine, coin purse hanging from his arm, stands next to the two women in green; perhaps they are family members who have hired medical men to carry out an autopsy on the deceased. Another man holding a book is positioned right next to the corpse and gestures to the bladder or public bone with a pointer. Since the ostensor's attention is on the lower abdomen, and there is no discernible genitalia, it is possible that this is another autopsy of a woman. Taking the

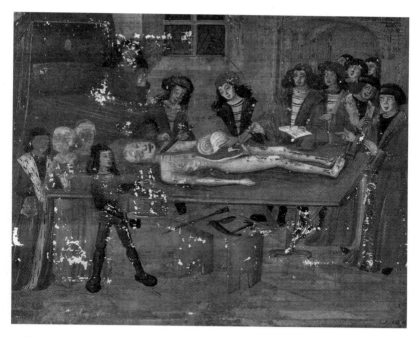

69 Dissection or autopsy, from Guy of Chauliac, *La grande chirurgie* (c. 1480–1500).

opportunity presented by a family agreeing to a post-mortem exploration of a cause of death to demonstrate the body's interior to students and other interested individuals certainly occurred. Indeed, accounts of private dissections occurring outside of the confines of those sanctioned by the universities are documented in Italy at this period (famously attended by artists such as Michelangelo in Florence) and were probably also taking place elsewhere.

A more straightforward late manuscript depiction of dissection appears in an incomplete, Latin copy of Avicenna's *Canon* made in Flanders in the late fifteenth century (Glasgow, University of Glasgow Library, MS Hunter 9).[17] Instead of presenting a single scene, the Glasgow manuscript features bodies in various stages of dissection, similar to Guido's images. Pictured in five column-width miniatures at the start of chapters describing individual organs, the corpses are in various stages of decomposition and not in Mondino dei Liuzzi's standard order of systematic dissection. At least one corpse is female. All five scenes are set outdoors, a group of men, richly dressed in robes trimmed in ermine, crowding around each plinth. The first miniature depicts an almost entirely decomposed skeleton, a black cavity for the abdomen and few discernible anatomical details. The second scene features a female corpse, breasts clearly visible, positioned at a diagonal across the frame, her head at lower left. Two surgeons lean over her body, one cutting into her upper right thigh, the other into her left wrist, both concentrating intently on their tasks as the spectators eagerly watch. The final three miniatures feature a similar composition, with a large group of men crowding around a central master who stands directly behind the horizontal dissection table. The first corpse is a skeleton, the second a partial skeleton pictured with organs still inside its abdominal cavity, and the third is an intact body, organs also displayed in the abdominal cavity (illus. 70). In each, the corpses' left hands are draped over their upper thighs. The organs visible in the interiors of the final two figures appear to be the heart, liver and spleen, connected by some blood vessels, above a rounded orb that could be the stomach.

It is notable that the Glasgow figures – some of the only manuscript versions after Guido to present different phases of cadaveric dissection – accompany the *Canon*, which does not describe the process of dissection, rather than Mondino's popular treatise. The dynamic and lively action of each miniature, their high level of decoration and the relative detail of the interiors render them particularly notable.

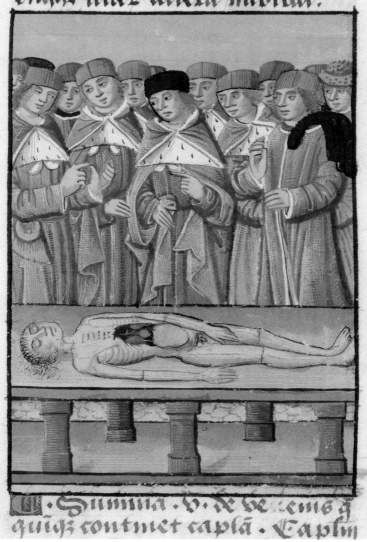

70 Dissection scene, from Avicenna, *Canon* (late 15th century).

Dissection in Incunabula

The earliest example of the dissection scene in a printed book is the 1482 Lyonnaise version of the *Livre des propriétés des choses* discussed earlier (see illus. 66). The positioning of the woodcut at the start of Book Five of Bartholomew's encyclopaedia recalls those images preceding anatomical texts written by medieval surgeons such as Mondino or Guy of Chauliac, in which one would expect the central figure to be a representation of the author. But Bartholomew's text does not mention human dissection. By beginning the book with a scene of dissection, it signalled to the reader that the text following would describe the parts of the body, regardless of the identity of the author of the work it accompanied. In this context, it represents the entire idea of anatomy, rather than prefiguring a description of human dissection.

Other dissection scenes soon cropped up outside of Mathieu Hutz's Lyonnaise printing circle.[18] Rather than presenting a group of students crowded together around a table, a German woodcut made to accompany an edition of Mondino's *Anathomia*, edited by the University of Leipzig medical professor Martin Pollich of Mellerstadt and printed in about 1493, only features two people besides the cadaver (illus. 71).[19] The professor is positioned above the action, literally and theoretically. He is seated in a *cathedra*, book open on his lap, gazing and gesturing to the foreground where a surgeon dissects a corpse. The surgeon looks back at him, listening to his instructions. The scene takes place outdoors, hills decorated with clusters of stubby trees and a rock formation. The separation between the professor, whose status as an established and learned man is heightened by his seated, hierarchically prominent position, and the lowly surgeon is here exaggerated to an extreme degree.

The pre-Vesalian printed dissection scene with the widest circulation, in the Italian translation of the *Fasciculus medicinae*

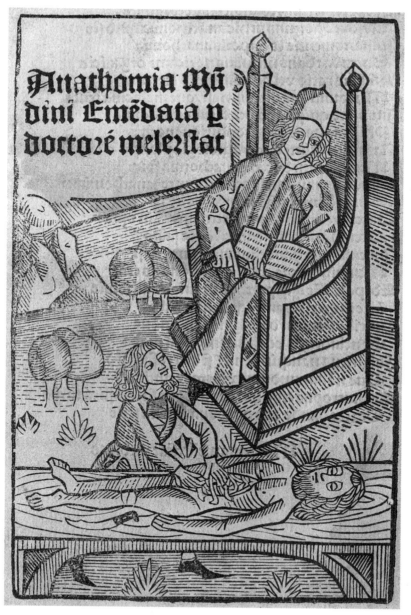

71 Dissection scene, title page woodcut of Mondino dei Liuzzi,
Anathomia (c. 1493).

(see illus. 65), likewise positions the lector high above the action of the dissection, but in an interior setting with a larger crowd, similar to what is seen in earlier manuscript and printed versions. The *Fasciculus medicinae* was the first printed medical manual to feature images as prominently as texts.[20] A slim volume containing six full-page drawings and their accompanying texts, the *Fasciculus* served as a general medical handbook, covering popular procedures like bloodletting and urinoscopy, as well as treatments for common diseases, illnesses and injuries. Printed by the brothers Giovanni and Gregorio de Gregori (or Johannes and Gregorius de Gregoriis) in Venice and edited by Giorgio dal Monferrato, the group of treatises are best known today as the '*Fasciculus medicinae* of Johannes de Ketham'. Despite the efforts of many to link this name to a historical figure, Johannes de Ketham's identity remains unknown, and to assign him ownership over the treatises gives the undue impression that he was their author, which is not true.[21] They were in most cases already several hundred years old by the end of the fifteenth century and attributed to medieval authors.

All six of the images in the initial print run of 1491 were taken from manuscript exemplars. Five of the six – the bloodletting man, zodiac man and Three-Figure Series (Disease Woman (illus. 33), Wound Man (illus. 31) and Disease Man) – have been discussed previously, and their components stayed largely the same during the transition to woodcut.[22] The compiler of the 1491 version most likely had access to either a manuscript with all six of these images and texts (for example, London, Wellcome MS 49; see illus. 31, 63), or to several manuscripts with the images and texts from which he compiled the 'little bundle'. In addition to being modelled themselves on manuscript images – perhaps most closely resembling in form and content those in Wellcome 49 – there is at least one definitive example of *Fasciculus* images being copied by manuscript

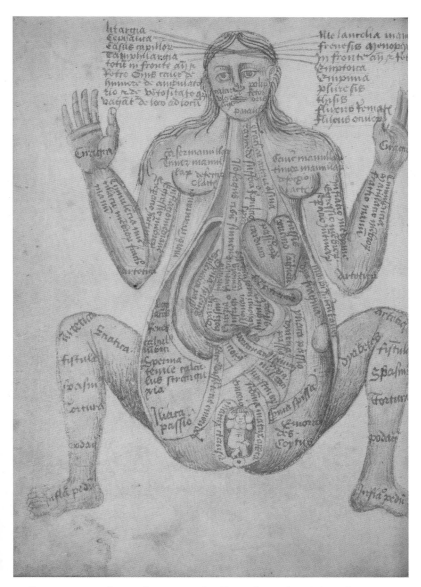

72 Disease woman, late 15th century, after *Fasciculus medicinae* (1491).

artists: London, Wellcome Library, MS 290. The Wellcome MS 290 Disease Woman (illus. 72) and Wound Man are shaded with cross-hatching, especially visible around their eyes, in imitation of the woodcut aesthetic.

About three years after it was originally printed, the *Fasciculus* was published in Italian as the *Fasciculo de medicina* and the figures were updated to reflect the type of idealized, anatomically proportional human form popularized by contemporary Italian artists (for example, see the Disease Woman evolution between illustrations 33 and 34).[23] Four new scenes of medical practice and two treatises were added, including the famous dissection scene prefacing Mondino's *Anathomia* (see illus. 65).[24] The *Fasciculo* dissection is in clear dialogue with the printed iconography established by the Lyon versions of the *Livre des propriétés des choses*. The lecturer is shown at a remove from the body being dissected, consulting a text (presumably, Mondino's) in an elaborate dais above the action, elegantly robed in an academic gown. He gestures as he looks straight ahead, in the midst of speaking, not looking down at the dissection, but rather directly at the viewer. Below the lectern is a crowded scene. The foreground is dominated by a large table upon which a male corpse rests. Several academics surround the body; some are paying attention to the dissection while others are in conversation, seemingly unconcerned with the action. The dissector bends over the body, making the first incision into the cadaver's sternum with a large knife. To his left, another man leans toward the corpse's head, gesturing to the corpse with a pointer. The dynamic action of the *Fasciculo* scene, juxtaposed with the positioning of the lecturer looking at the viewer rather than engaging with the other figures, lends a performative and self-consciously important bent to the image. The central significance of the lecturer is highlighted by his positioning; although the dissector below is performing the act, the lecturer is the protagonist. His prominence tells the viewer that his repetition of established theories about the body is the most important part of the scene.

* * *

By the time Vesalius published the *Fabrica* in 1543, anatomy was experiencing a surge in popularity in both art and medicine, becoming an interdisciplinary field of knowledge that was critically important for both artists and physicians to master. Most medical faculties in Europe had professorships in anatomy, positions only created at the end of the fifteenth century. As explored in the previous chapter, artists began to insert themselves into medical practice by attending dissections and incorporating what they saw into their own works, and they were increasingly focused on depicting human anatomy as accurately (albeit idealistically) as possible.

Contemporary medical texts published by Vesalius's peers contained anatomical sections, some illustrated, but Vesalius chose to elevate his illustrations to be as important – if not more so – than his text itself, inviting art into academic anatomy instead of what had until then mostly been the adoption of academic anatomy by artists. When considered in conjunction with his 'competitors', Vesalius's *Fabrica*, with its hundreds of detailed illustrations of the interior, for which he recruited professional artists from the studio of famed Venetian painter Titian (d. 1576), did indeed represent a significant departure from the norm.[25] Although some of his contemporaries, like Jacopo Berengario of Carpi, included their own imagery in their anatomical treatises (see illus. 62), none were as painstakingly and copiously illustrated, and none featured scenes of the author performing dissection himself. With the publication of the *Fabrica*, anatomy was cemented as critically important to medicine and art, a pursuit of important truths only achievable by exploration through human dissection. And, as Vesalius's frontispiece would have his viewers believe, such truths could only be discoverable by an individual able to work despite the noise of the 'squawking jackdaws' chained by the oppressive weight of tradition.

However, as has been demonstrated here, Vesalius's characterizations of the act of dissection and the radicalness of his own achievements were not entirely accurate. Indeed, his use of the dissection scene as his frontispiece was already an established tradition in anatomical treatises, both manuscript and print. In addition, Guido of Vigevano had himself pictured as boldly as Vesalius did, the graphic centre of the process of dissection, two centuries earlier, and argued just as convincingly for the usefulness of images for anatomical study. And despite Vesalius's implication that he was the first anatomist to actually perform human dissection with his own hands, the influential Mondino dei Liuzzi's work proved otherwise. As Mondino wrote in the preface to his anatomical manual, 'I shall not adopt an elevated style, but shall merely seek to convey such knowledge as manual practice requires.'[26] He and his fellow medieval surgeons at the University of Bologna performed human dissection when there was no direct precedent; they believed they were following in Galen's footsteps, when in reality, even Galen had not ventured to dissect human beings. Their adoption of human cadaveric dissection should thus be considered the more radical break from tradition than Vesalius's achievements, important though they were. But through his manipulation of existing anatomical practices and imagery, Vesalius was able to shape perception of himself as a radical. As has been proven in this chapter and indeed this whole work, however, Vesalius's achievements cannot be fully celebrated without recognizing the daring medieval surgeons whose earlier efforts outside the bounds of their textual and artistic confines paved the way for him to reach such heights.

Conclusion

This exploration of medieval European anatomical illustration has shown the wide variety of visual modes used to express anatomical theories and the makers who considered these images useful for learning and instruction or as decoration. While the point of this book has been to celebrate these differences, there are a few collective takeaways that can be discerned in the composition, form and function of anatomical images made during the Middle Ages.

First, the images can be divided into two general visual styles: diagrammatic and narrative. Broadly, the diagrammatic used text and image to communicate ideas and instruct practitioners and students, while the narrative indicated the overall value of anatomy in medical treatment.

Within the diagrammatic tradition, the images can be further separated into two graphic types: the use of the full body as a template onto which anatomy was transposed, and those that featured anatomical elements on their own, outside the familiar bounds of the flesh. The first grouping is by far the largest, comprising both early medieval (and even likely pre-medieval) and related non-Western images in which different systems, like the veins or bones, were patterned on the repeated shape of the living, 'X-rayed' human form. These types of graphics drew upon the communal experience of the body as a starting point: one can easily understand that the liver is positioned over the

stomach on the right side of the abdomen, for instance, and
know its relative size and shape. But the purpose of medieval
anatomcal imagery was not to communicate the way in which
the organs fit together within the body; rather, it sought to convey the function of each part, both alone and together with the
other parts in a system. By breaking down the information into
different systems – comprising the simple and the compound
– each could be examined and digested on its own without the
confusing overlay of different parts, so that one could better
understand the fundamentals of Galenic physiology. The images
themselves also offered viewpoints that could not be easily seen
in real-life dissections – uncommon though they were.

The full body also served as the graphic foundation for more
theoretical medicine, especially the relationship between the
parts of the body and exterior factors. These connections ranged
from the movements of the stars and planets to the more mundane questions of what to eat and when. Diagrams of these ideas
often superimposed zodiac signs on their related body parts or
drew lines extending from explicatory text blocks to point out
different veins for bloodletting to regulate the humours. The
understanding of the wellness and function of the body as reliant
on these exterior factors was fundamental to medical treatment,
and these images served to both communicate these ideas as
well as aid a practitioner in treatment.

The second type of diagrammatic anatomical figure presented elements of interior anatomy outside of the context of
the body. Illustratively, this was done either through geometric
abstraction designed to communicate physiological processes,
or through static exterior depictions of organs as they might generally appear in life. Many of the former were devised to convey
function rather than form, and those functions had to be clarified through captions and brief descriptions within the image.
Descriptions were often necessary for the simplified exterior

views, as well, but for different reasons; their form was so basic that they were sometimes unidentifiable.

The second grouping of medieval anatomical images, narrative scenes, featured the performance of dissection rather than drawing upon diagrams of already dissected bodies or organs, and thereby emphasized humanistic agency within the fields of anatomy and surgery. As early as the thirteenth century, professional workshop artists produced miniatures and historiated initials of dissected bodies to punctuate anatomical texts. In the early fourteenth century, the effect of the establishment of human dissection in medical curricula led to the dissectors themselves adding visual aids to their manuals. The first unambiguous representation of cadaveric dissection came in the mid-fourteenth century by one of these surgeon-authors, Guido of Vigevano, who had himself depicted as the dissector. By the middle of the next century, as the practice of human dissection swelled in university medical curricula across western Europe, scenes representing the practice were introduced in most illustrated medical texts. In these images, the physicians and surgeons played their individual parts, generally watched by an audience, which both stands in for the viewer and lends a sense of importance to the process of dissection. The power of such images lay not in showing the viewer pictures of internal anatomy, but rather in emphasizing the significance of the study of anatomy and medicine in general – not only within the bounds of university medicine, but for artists who began to observe internal anatomy for their own graphic purposes. Anatomists increasingly enlisted artists skilled in depicting anatomy to illustrate their treatises.

How can we understand this range of diverse illustrative forms within the broader scope of medieval medicine and medieval art? The short answer is there is no easy way to do so. The imagery discussed here – mostly confined, as discussed in the introduction, to figures that were devised to accompany medical writings – are a small corpus of visual materials in comparison to other medieval textual illustrations, like those accompanying books of hours. Some anatomical figures circulated through monastic houses, some through surgical treatises, some had a wider audience through printing. Some were made without the input of professional artists, drawn by monks in monastic scriptoria as supplements to divine contemplation. Many of the images did not reflect an understanding of or engagement with contemporary artistic movements or fashions, while others prioritized those considerations over conveying physiological theories.

In the end, the rich variety of graphic approaches speaks to the many creative ways in which people of the medieval period tried to understand the mysteries of the body. And, as is the case in contemporary medicine, there is no one way to illustrate anatomy. A plastic (or real) skeleton hangs in high school biology classrooms around the world; a Google search of any anatomical feature will turn up photographs of the part of varying quality, neat and organized illustrations of causes and effects, computer-generated models, X-rays, MRI scans or flow charts explaining functions. Each of these visual aids contributes to medical training and practice in different and equally meaningful ways. The fact that so many different medieval makers tried their hand at creating visual accompaniments for anatomical texts speaks to the enduring usefulness of didactic imagery in even so nebulous and dynamic a field in medieval thought as anatomy.

REFERENCES

Introduction

1 For a recent definition and discussion of diagrams, especially in medieval manuscripts, see Jeffrey F. Hamburger, *Diagramming Devotion: Berthold of Nuremberg's Transformation of Hrabanus Maurus's 'Poems in Praise of the Cross'* (Chicago, IL, 2020), esp. pp. 13–32.

2 Michael McVaugh articulates the major differences between medieval and contemporary anatomy by defining the medieval as 'two dimensional', concerned with function above form, versus contemporary 'three-dimensional' anatomy, in which the actual physical organization of the parts within the body is the focus; see Michael McVaugh, 'Fistulas, the Knee, and the "Three-Dimensional" Body', in *Medicine and Space: Body, Surroundings and Borders in Antiquity and the Middle Ages*, ed. Patricia A. Baker, Han Nijdam and Karine van't Land (Leiden and Boston, MA, 2012), pp. 23–36, at pp. 23–4.

3 For the most up-to-date in-depth treatment of medieval anatomical diagrams, see Taylor McCall, 'Illuminating the Interior: The Illustrations of the Nine Systems of the Body and Anatomical Knowledge in Medieval Europe', PhD diss., University of Cambridge, 2017. A list of the most important treatments of medieval anatomical imagery must begin with Karl Sudhoff's oeuvre, including most notably 'Anatomische Zeichnungen (Schemata) aus dem 12. und 13. Jahrhundert und eine Skelettzeichnung des 14. Jahrhunderts', *Studien zur Geschichte der Medizin*, I (1907), pp. 49–65; *Ein Beitrag zur Geschichte der Anatomie im Mittelalter speziell der anatomischen Graphik nach Handschriften des 9. bis 15. Jahrhunderts* (Leipzig, 1908; repr. Hildesheim, 1964); *Weitere Beiträge zur Geschichte der Anatomie im Mittelalter, Archiv für Geschichte der Medizin*, VIII (Leipzig, 1914); and *Beiträge zur Geschichte der Chirurgie im Mittelalter, graphische und textliche Untersuchungen in mittelalterlichen Handschriften*, 2 vols (Leipzig, 1914–18). General overviews of medieval medical imagery include Loren C. MacKinney's *Medical Illustrations in Medieval Manuscripts* (London, 1965); and Peter Murray Jones's *Medieval Medicine in Illuminated Manuscripts*, 2nd edn (London,

1998). Larger histories of anatomy that have useful sections on the medieval period are Ludwig Choulant, *History and Bibliography of Anatomic Illustration*, trans. Mortimer Frank (Chicago, IL, 1920); Robert Herrlinger, *History of Medical Illustration from Antiquity to AD 1600* (Nijkerk, 1970); John E. Murdoch, *Album of Science: Antiquity and the Middle Ages* (New York, 1984); and Loris Premuda, *Storia dell'iconografia anatomica* (Milan, 1957).

4 Phaidon Editors, *Anatomy: Exploring the Human Body* (London, 2019). The word 'anatomy' combines the Greek words *temnein*, 'to cut', with *ana*, meaning 'up', to form what literally means 'to cut up'.

5 A selection of the many important studies addressing the depiction of bodies in the Middle Ages relevant to this study include Caroline Walker Bynum, 'Why All the Fuss About the Body? A Medievalist's Perspective', *Critical Inquiry*, XX/1 (1995), pp. 1–33; Joan Cadden, *Meanings of Sex Difference in the Middle Ages: Medicine, Science, and Culture* (Cambridge, 1993); Linda Kalof, ed., *A Cultural History of the Human Body in the Medieval Age* (Oxford, 2010); Sarah Kay and Miri Rubin, eds, *Framing Medieval Bodies* (Manchester, 1994); and Caroline Walker Bynum, *Fragmentation and Redemption: Essays on Gender and the Human Body in Medieval Religion* (New York, 1990). For studies focusing on the queer experience and representations, see Robert Mills, *Seeing Sodomy in the Middle Ages* (Chicago, IL, 2015); and Glenn Burger and Steven Kruger, eds, *Queering the Middle Ages* (Minneapolis, MN, 2001). Michael Camille focused much of his discussion of marginalia on depictions of sodomy, as well as bodies generally, in *Image on the Edge: The Margins of Medieval Art* [1992] (London, 2008).

6 Peter Murray Jones has discussed the complicated relationships between medical images and texts in manuscripts in 'Image, Word, and Medicine in the Middle Ages', in *Visualizing Medieval Medicine and Natural History, 1200–1550*, ed. Jean A. Givens, Karen Reeds and Alain Touwaide (Aldershot, 2006), pp. 1–24.

7 Emile Littré, *Oeuvres complètes d'Hippocrate: Traduction nouvelle avec le texte grec en regard*, 10 vols (Paris, 1839–61; repr. Amsterdam, 1961–2). For more on the Hippocratic corpus, see Pearl Kibre, *Hippocrates Latinus: Repertorium of Hippocratic Writings in the Latin Middle Ages* (New York, 1985); and on classical medicine in general, *Oxford Handbook of Science and Medicine in the Classical World*, ed. Paul T. Keyser and John Scarborough (New York and Oxford, 2018).

8 Aristotle's detailed descriptions of animal anatomy indicating dissection are found in (among others) his *History of Animals*,

On the Motion of Animals and *On the Parts of Animals*; see *The Complete Works of Aristotle*, vols I and II, ed. Jonathan Barnes (Princeton, NJ, 1994).

9 In *History of Animals*, Book I, Chapter 17, for example, Aristotle describes the female womb and references a figure: 'All the parts mentioned are similar in the female as well; there is no difference so far as the internal parts are concerned, except for the uterus, the appearance of which should be studied in the diagram in the *Dissections*' (Aristotle, *History of Animals*, vol. I: *Books 1–3*, trans. A. L. Peck (Cambridge, MA, 1965)).

10 Heinrich von Staden, *Herophilus: The Art of Medicine in Early Alexandria* [1989] (Cambridge, 2007).

11 R. J. Hankinson, ed., *The Cambridge Companion to Galen* (Cambridge, 2008); and Vivian Nutton, *Ancient Medicine*, 2nd edn (London, 2013), esp. pp. 222–53. Roger French provides a useful overview of the reception of Galen's anatomical writings in '*De juvamentis membrorum* and the Reception of Galenic Physiological Anatomy', *Isis*, LXX (1979), pp. 96–109.

12 Peter E. Pormann and Emilie Savage-Smith, *Medieval Islamic Medicine* (Edinburgh, 2007); and Danielle Jacquart and Françoise Micheau, *La médecine arabe et l'occident médiéval* (Paris, 1990).

13 Byzantine medical manuscripts are mostly unillustrated and therefore do not make much of an appearance here. For a recent treatment of medical texts in Byzantium and a related bibliography see Petros Bouras-Vallianatos, 'Cross-Cultural Transfer of Medical Knowledge in the Medieval Mediterranean: The Introduction and Dissemination of Sugar-Based Potions from the Islamic World to Byzantium', *Speculum*, CXLIV/4 (2021), pp. 963–1008.

14 A. Mark Smith, *From Sight to Light: The Passage from Ancient to Modern Optics* (Chicago, IL, 2014), esp. pp. 181–224.

15 Emilie Savage-Smith, 'Anatomical Illustration in Arabic Manuscripts', in *Arab Painting: Text and Image in Illustrated Arabic Manuscripts*, ed. Anna Contadini (Leiden, 2007), pp. 147–59.

16 This illustration is found in a 1083 (15 Jumādā I 476) copy of the *Kitab al-Manazir*, now in Istanbul's Süleimaniye Mosque Library, MS Fatih 3212, vol. I, fol. 81b. See Savage-Smith, 'Anatomical Illustration in Arabic Manuscripts', pp. 148–55.

17 Monica H. Green, 'Medical Books', in *The European Book in the Twelfth Century*, ed. Erik Kwakkel and Rodney Thomson (Cambridge, 2018), pp. 277–92, at pp. 284–5.

18 This manuscript, known as the Vienna Dioscorides (Österreichische
Nationalbibliothek, Medicus Graecus 1), was created in about
512 for the daughter of the emperor Flavius Anicius Olybrius,
Anicia Juliana. It contains more than five hundred illustrations
of plants and animals. For more on the herbal tradition, see Anne
Van Arsdall and Timothy Graham, eds, *Herbs and Healers from the
Ancient Mediterranean through the Medieval West: Essays in Honor of
John M. Riddle* (Farnham, 2012).

19 Florence, Biblioteca Medica Laurenziana, MS Plut. 73.41, includes
a tenth-century copy of sixteen cautery images that were inserted at
the end of a ninth-century medical compendium.

20 Muscio's *Gynaecia* was based on the well-known gynaecological
and obstetrical writings by Soranus of Ephesus (second century
CE). For more on the images associated with Muscio and Soranus,
see Francesca Marchetti, 'Educating the Midwife: The Role of
Illustrations in Late Antique and Medieval Obstetrical Texts', in
*Pregnancy and Childbirth in the Premodern World: European and Middle
Eastern Cultures, from Late Antiquity to the Renaissance*, ed. Costanza
Gislon Dopfel, Alessandra Foscati and Charles Burnett (Turnhout,
2019), pp. 3–28.

21 This is not to say they could not have been; see, for example,
Alison Beach's study of female scribes active in the same area
and time period in which Clm 13002 was produced: Alison I.
Beach, *Women as Scribes: Book Production and Monastic Reform in
Twelfth-Century Bavaria* (Cambridge, 2004). For a recent discussion
of medicine and illustrated medical texts made for and with the
input of women outside of the monastery, see Jennifer Borland,
*Visualizing Household Health: Medieval Women, Art, and Knowledge
in the 'Régime du corps'* (University Park, PA, 2022). For more on
women and medicine in the Middle Ages in general, specifically
the exclusion of women from access to learned medical texts
available to monks and male medical students and practitioners,
see Monica H. Green, *Women's Healthcare in the Medieval West:
Texts and Contexts* (Burlington, VT, 2000), especially 'The
Possibilities of Literacy and the Limits of Reading: Women and
the Gendering of Medical Literacy', pp. 1–76; and Monica
H. Green, *Making Women's Medicine Masculine: The Rise of
Male Authority in Pre-Modern Gynecology* (Oxford, 2008).

22 Carmen Caballero-Navas, 'Medicine among Medieval Jews:
The Science, the Art, and the Practice', in *Science in Medieval
Jewish Cultures*, ed. Gad Freudenthal (Cambridge, 2011),

pp. 320–42; and Joseph Shatzmiller, *Jews, Medicine, and Medieval Society* (Berkeley, CA, 1994).

23 The broader field of medieval studies has been grappling with issues of race and racism. Two of many recent important studies on the topic are Geraldine Heng, *The Invention of Race in the European Middle Ages* (Cambridge, 2018); and Cord J. Whitaker, *Black Metaphors: How Modern Racism Emerged from Medieval Race-Thinking* (Philadelphia, PA, 2019). For an up-to-date account of the engagement of medieval art history with depictions of race, including extensive bibliography on race and racism in medieval art, see Pamela A. Patton, 'What Did Medieval Slavery Look Like? Color, Race, and Unfreedom in Later Medieval Iberia', *Speculum*, XCVII/3 (2022), pp. 649–97, esp. pp. 650–51, nn. 2–4.

24 These were part of Mansūr ibn Muḥammad ibn Amād ibn Yūsuf ibn Ilyās's (*fl.* 1380–1420) *Tashrīḥ-i badan-i insān* (Anatomy of the Human Body).

25 For more on the differences between men and women, see Cadden, *Meanings of Sex Difference*, esp. pp. 170–80.

1 Spiritual Anatomy and the Monastery

1 Elisabeth Klemm, *Die romanischen Handschriften der Bayerischen Staatsbibliothek*, Teil 1: *Die Bistümer Regensburg, Passau und Salzburg, Katalog der illuminierten Handschriften der Bayerischen Staatsbibliothek in München 3*, 2 vols (Wiesbaden, 1980), pp. 160–64 and 150–64; Elisabeth Klemm, 'Die Regensburger Buchmalerei des 12. Jahrhunderts', in *Regensburger Buchmalerei: Von frühkarolingischer Zeit bis zum Ausgang des Mittelalters* (Munich, 1987), pp. 40–42 and 50; and Melanie Holcomb, ed., *Pen and Parchment: Drawing in the Middle Ages* (New York, 2009), pp. 91–3.

2 'Five-Figure Series' is a translation of the German *Fünfbilderserie*, the term bestowed upon the images by Karl Sudhoff, who first discussed them in detail; see *Ein Beitrag zur Geschichte der Anatomie im Mittelalter speziell der anatomischen Graphik nach Handschriften des 9. bis 15. Jahrhunderts* (Leipzig, 1908; repr. Hildesheim, 1964); for more recent scholarship, see Taylor McCall, 'Illuminating the Interior: The Illustrations of the Nine Systems of the Body and Anatomical Knowledge in Medieval Europe', PhD diss., University of Cambridge, 2017.

3 Adam Cohen, 'Making Memories in a Medieval Miscellany', in *Making Thoughts, Making Pictures, Making Memories in Late Antiquity*

and the Middle Ages: Essays in Honor of Mary Carruthers, ed. Anne
D. Hedeman, *Gesta*, XLVIII/2 (2009), pp. 135–52.

4 For recent examinations of these and many other types of diagrams,
see Marcia Kupfer, Adam S. Cohen and J. H. Chajes, eds, *The
Visualization of Knowledge in Medieval and Early Modern Europe*
(Turnhout, 2020), especially the contributions by Barbara Obrist
('The Idea of a Spherical Universe and Its Visualization in the
Earlier Middle Ages [Seventh to Twelfth Century]', pp. 229–58);
Marcia Kupfer ('The Rhetoric of World Maps in Late Antiquity and
the Middle Ages', pp. 259–90); and Adam S. Cohen ('Diagramming
the Diagrammatic: Twelfth-Century Europe', pp. 383–404).

5 Clm 13002, fol. 2v. Karl Sudhoff was the first to transcribe and
publish the *Historia incisionis* text from the Prüfening manuscript in
'Abermals eine neue Handschrift der anatomischen Fünfbilderserie',
Archiv für Geschichte der Medizin, III (1910), pp. 353–68.

6 Cohen, 'Making Memories', p. 141.

7 Although he was referring to sick members of the monastic
community, many monks served local people as well. '22.
Medical Injunctions in the *Rule of St Benedict*', in *Medieval
Medicine: A Reader*, ed. Faith Wallis (Toronto, 2010), pp. 82–4.
For an overview of monastic medicine during the period in
question, see Elma Brenner, 'The Medical Role of Monasteries
in the Latin West, *c.* 1050–1300', in *The Cambridge History of
Medieval Monasticism in the Latin West*, ed. Alison I. Beach and
Isabelle Cochelin (Cambridge, 2020), pp. 865–81.

8 Adam J. Davis, *The Medieval Economy of Salvation: Charity,
Commerce, and the Rise of the Hospital* (Ithaca, NY, 2019).

9 Cassiodorus, *Institutiones*, Book I, Chapter 30, trans. James
W. Halporn and Barbara Halporn, available online via Georgetown
University: https://faculty.georgetown.edu, accessed 26 June 2020.

10 See, for instance, the case of the Winchester Bible, upon which
at least six different professional illuminators worked, as first
explored by Walter Oakeshott in *The Artists of the Winchester
Bible* (London, 1945).

11 The most up-to-date account of Constantine's life is Eliza Glaze,
'Introduction: Constantine the African and the *Pantegni* in
Context', in Erik Kwakkel and Francis Newton, *Medicine at Monte
Cassino: Constantine the African and the Oldest Manuscript of his
'Pantegni'* (Turnhout, 2019), pp. 1–29. For more on Constantine
and his work, see Kwakkel and Newton, *Medicine at Monte Cassino*,
and the *Constantinus Africanus* blog edited by Monica H. Green

and Brian Long: https://constantinusafricanus.com, accessed
13 June 2021.

12 Ynez Violé O'Neill, 'The *Fünfbilderserie* Reconsidered', *Bulletin of
the History of Medicine*, xliii/3 (1969), pp. 236–45. Philip de Lacey's
1981 English translation of the *De placitis Hippocratis et Platonis* is
available online at http://cmg.bbaw.de, accessed 13 June 2021.

13 I am very grateful to Monica H. Green, who has done extensive
work on Constantine and his oeuvre, for first pointing this out
to me; see Monica H. Green, 'Richard de Fournival and the
Reconfiguration of Learned Medicine in the 13th Century', in
Richard de Fournival et les sciences au xiiie siècle, ed. Joëlle Ducos
and Christopher Lucken (Florence, 2018), pp. 179–206, at p. 203.

14 Fritz Saxl, 'A Spiritual Encyclopaedia of the Later Middle
Ages', *Journal of the Courtauld and Warburg Institutes*, v (1942),
pp. 82–137.

15 Cohen, 'Making Memories', pp. 135–52.

16 The microfilm of bsb, Clm 17403 is digitized: urn:nbn:de:bvb:
12-bsb00110824-7. See the catalogue description for more
bibliography.

17 The entire Five-Figure Series and *Historia incisionis* appears in a
manuscript in the Czech Republic (Nelahozeves Castle, Roudnice
Lobkowicz Library, ms vi Fc 29), which was probably produced in
the late fourteenth century in Bohemia. Two Italian manuscripts
include just the five figures, uncoloured and unlabelled (Oxford,
Bodleian Library, ms e Mus. 19 (late thirteenth century); and Milan,
Trivulziana Library, ms 836 (mid-fourteenth century)). Dresden's
Sächsische Landesbibliothek, ms c.310 (completed 1323, possibly
in Germany), is unique in that it only includes the first four out of
the five sections of the *Historia incisionis* text and just one unlabelled
figure, a fleshless, grinning skeleton that looks exceedingly different
to the other versions of the bone system.

18 For a discussion of the fifteenth-century medical miscellany of
Gonville and Caius College, ms 190/223, see Peter Murray Jones,
'*Experimenta*, Compilation and Construction in Two Medieval
Books', *Poetica: An International Journal of Linguistic-Literary Studies*,
xci and xcii (2019), pp. 61–80.

19 Catalogue treatments of Gonville and Caius ms 190/223 include
M. R. James, *A Descriptive Catalogue of the Manuscripts in the
Library of Gonville and Caius College*, vol. 1 (Cambridge, 1907), no.
190/223 and Paul Binski and Stella Panayotova, eds, *The Cambridge
Illuminations: Ten Centuries of Book Production in the Medieval West*

(Cambridge, 2005), no. 154. For further bibliography, see Taylor
McCall, 'Reliquam dicit pictura: Text and Image in an Illustrated
Anatomical Manual (Gonville and Caius MS 190/223)', Transactions
of the Cambridge Bibliographical Society, XVI/1 (2016), pp. 1–22; the
images are also treated in detail in Taylor McCall, 'Functional
Abstraction in Medieval Anatomical Diagrams', in Abstraction
in Medieval Art: Beyond the Ornament, ed. Elina Gertsman
(Amsterdam, 2021), pp. 285–308.

20 These examples will be discussed in more detail presently, but the
other two manuscripts with the entire nine figures are Oxford,
Bodleian Library, MS Ashmole 399 and London, Wellcome Library,
MS 49, and the organ diagrams alone are found in a booklet now in
two pieces: the first is Pisa, Universitaria Biblioteca, MS 735, and
the second is in a private collection in Switzerland.

21 See Peter Murray Jones, 'Image, Word, and Medicine in the
Middle Ages', in Visualizing Medieval Medicine and Natural History,
1200–1550, ed. Jean A. Givens, Karen Reeds and Alain Touwaide
(Aldershot, 2006), pp. 1–24; and Gertsman, ed., Abstraction in
Medieval Art.

22 For more on the use of abstraction in medieval anatomy, see
McCall, 'Functional Abstraction'.

23 McCall, 'Reliquam dicit pictura'.

24 The few detailed descriptions of the male genitalia as it appears
in the Nine-Figure Series can be found in Charles Singer, 'Note
on a Thirteenth Century Diagram of the Male Genitalia',
Studies in the History and Method of Science, I (1917), pp. 212–14;
Christoph Ferckel, 'Diagramme der sexualorgane in mittelalterliche
Handschriften', Archiv für Geschichte der Medizin, X (1917),
pp. 255–63; and Carlo Maccagni, 'Frammento di un codice di
medicina del secolo XIV (manoscritto N. 735. già codice Roncioni
N. 99) della Biblioteca Universitaria di Pisa', Physis, XI (1969),
pp. 311–78.

25 Karl Whittington, 'The Cruciform Womb: Process, Symbol and
Salvation in Bodleian Library MS. Ashmole 399', Different Visions:
A Journal of New Perspectives on Medieval Art, I (2008), pp. 1–24,
available at https://differentvisions.org.

26 Aristotle describes the bicornate uterus in the History of Animals I,
Ch. 17 and in III, Ch. 1, where he refers to a diagram of a bicornate
uterus in his now-lost work Anatomy. See also Katharine Park,
Secrets of Women: Gender, Generation, and the Origins of Human
Dissection (New York, 2010), pp. 114, 184–5, 339, n. 68.

27 Aristotle downplayed the importance of the brain, arguing that
   the heart was both the seat of all sensations and controlled the
   movement of the parts of the body; see *On the Parts of Animals*,
   trans. A. L. Peck and E. S. Forster (Cambridge, MA, 1965),
   Book II, Chapter 10. Galen disagreed with Aristotle, concluding
   that the brain was in fact responsible for all sensation, mental
   faculties and movement; see Julius Rocca, *Galen on the Brain:
   Anatomical Knowledge and Physiological Speculation in the Second
   Century A.D.* (Leiden, 2003), especially Chs 5 and 6.

28 Ynez Violé O'Neill, 'Diagrams of the Medieval Brain', in
   Iconography at the Crossroads, ed. Brendan Cassidy (Princeton,
   NJ, 1990), pp. 91–105; and Ynez Violé O'Neill, 'Meningeal
   Localization: A New Key to Some Medical Texts, Diagrams
   and Practices of the Middle Ages', *Mediaevistik*, VI (1993),
   pp. 211–38. Diagrams of the eye alone sometimes accompany
   treatises on optics.

29 For more on diagrams of the mind, see Mary Carruthers, 'Two
   Unusual Mind Diagrams in a Late Fifteenth-Century Manuscript
   (UPenn Schoenberg Collection, MS LJS 429)', *Manuscript Studies:
   A Journal of the Schoenberg Institute for Manuscript Studies*, IV (2019),
   pp. 389–400, as well as more general overviews in Annemieke
   R. Verboon, 'Brain Ventricle Diagrams: A Century after Walther
   Sudhoff; New Manuscript Sources from the XVth Century', *Sudhoffs
   Archiv*, XCVIII (2014), pp. 212–33; and Edwin Clarke and Kenneth
   Dewhurst, *An Illustrated History of Brain Function* (Oxford, 1972).

30 Taylor McCall, 'Disembodied: Additional MS. 8785 and the Tradition
   of Human Organ Depictions in Medieval Art and Medicine',
   Electronic British Library Journal (2018), article 8, pp. 1–26, at
   pp. 17–19, http://vll-minos.bl.uk, accessed 7 October 2022; and
   McCall, 'Illuminating the Interior', pp. 63–5.

31 James G. Clark, 'Monks and the Universities, *c.* 1200–1500', in
   The Cambridge History of Medieval Monasticism, ed. Beach and
   Cochelin, pp. 1074–92.

32 Gregor Maurach, 'Johannicius. *Isagoge ad Techne Galieni*', *Sudhoffs
   Archiv*, LXII (1978), pp. 148–74.

33 For more on the lasting impact of the *Articella*, see Jon Arrizabalaga,
   The 'Articella' in the Early Press, c. 1476–1534 (Cambridge, 1998).

34 For an overview of the establishment of medical faculty in medieval
   Europe, see Nancy G. Siraisi, *Medieval and Early Renaissance
   Medicine: An Introduction to Knowledge and Practice* (Chicago, IL,
   1990), esp. Ch. 3, 'Medical Education', pp. 48–77.

35 Fragments or sketches of the Five-Figure Series likely made in
university settings are those in Oxford, Bodleian Library, MS e
Mus. 19 (late thirteenth century) and Milan, Trivulziana Library,
MS 836 (mid-fourteenth century), both of which are Italian, as well
as Dresden's Sächsische Landesbibliothek, MS c.310 (completed
1323, possibly in Germany). The textual components of these three
manuscripts are miscellaneous medical treatises popular with students.

36 See Maccagni, 'Frammento', pp. 311–78, for the most detailed
description of the Pisa manuscript. The Swiss fragment was
unknown until it was sold by Sotheby's London in 1997 ('Cautery,
a Bifolium on Vellum from an Illustrated Medical Manuscript',
in Western Manuscripts and Miniatures, 2 December 1997 (sales
catalogue), London: Sotheby's and Co., 2 December 1997, lot 36,
pp. 38–41) and has only been discussed in McCall, 'Illuminating
the Interior', pp. 88–93.

37 Christopher de Hamel initially judged the script to be from the
second quarter of the thirteenth century ('Cautery, a Bifolium on
Vellum', p. 38) and reconfirmed his opinion in private correspond-
ence (November 2014). He also cites 'Italy (possibly Sicily)' as the
place of creation in his catalogue description of the Swiss fragment.

38 M. B. Parkes, 'The Hereford Map: The Handwriting and Copying
of the Text', in The Hereford World Map: Medieval World Maps and
Their Context, ed. P.D.A. Harvey (London, 2006), pp. 107–9.

39 Nigel Morgan, 'Hereford Map: Art-Historical Aspects', in The
Hereford World Map, ed. Harvey, pp. 119–36, at pp. 123–4; and
Lucy Freeman Sandler, Gothic Manuscripts, 1285–1385, 2 vols, in
A Survey of Manuscripts Illuminated in the British Isles, v (London,
1986), vol. I, pp. 41–42; vol. II, no. 19, p. 28.

40 See especially Angela Montford, Health, Sickness, Medicine and the
Friars in the Thirteenth and Fourteenth Centuries (Aldershot, 2004).

41 Almuth Seebohm, Apokalypse, ars moriendi, medizinische Traktate,
Tugend- und Lasterlehren: die erbaulich-didaktische Sammelhandschrift
London, Wellcome Institute for the History of Medicine, Ms. 49
(Munich, 1995); and Saxl, 'A Spiritual Encyclopaedia', pp. 82–137,
followed by an appendix by Otto Kurtz, 'Appendix II: The Medical
Illustrations', pp. 137–42. See also Boyd H. Hill Jr, 'Another Member
of the Sudhoff Fünfbilderserie – Wellcome MS 5000', Sudhoffs Archiv
fur Geschichte der Medezin un der Naturwissenchaften, 43 (1959),
pp. 13–19; Hill, 'The Fünfbilderserie', pp. 143–69; and Boyd H. Hill
Jr, 'A Medieval German Wound Man: Wellcome MS 49', Journal of
the History of Medicine and Allied Sciences, XX/4 (1965), pp. 334–57.

42 Saxl, 'A Spiritual Encyclopaedia', pp. 116–17 and 117–25. Monica
   H. Green also considers the inclusion of gynaecological subjects
   alongside religious materials in manuscripts created for male owners
   in *Making Women's Medicine Masculine: The Rise of Male Authority in
   Pre-Modern Gynecology* (Oxford, 2008), esp. pp. 157–9.

2 Blood and Stars: Anatomical Astrology

1 Ancient cultures worldwide connected man's physical presence
  on Earth to the movements of the planets and the stars; see *Astro-
  Medicine: Astrology and Medicine, East and West*, ed. Anna Akasoy,
  Charles Burnett and Ronit Yoeli-Tlalim (Florence, 2008); and
  Markham Judah Geller, *Melothesia in Babylonia: Medicine, Magic,
  and Astrology in the Ancient Near East* (Berlin, Boston, MA, and
  Munich, 2014).
2 For an overview of astrology and medicine in the western Middle
  Ages, see Roger French, 'Astrology in Medical Practice', in *Practical
  Medicine from Salerno to the Black Death*, ed. Luis García-Ballester,
  Roger French, Jon Arrizabalaga and Andrew Cunningham
  (Cambridge, 1994), pp. 30–59.
3 Conrad Rudolph, 'Macro/Microcosm at Vézelay: The Narthex
  Portal and Non-Elite Participation in Elite Spirituality', *Speculum*,
  XCVI/3 (2021): pp. 601–61, at pp. 616–20.
4 Martin Kauffman, 'Decoration and Illustration', in *The European
  Book in the Twelfth Century*, ed. Erik Kwakkel and Rodney Thomson
  (Cambridge, 2018), pp. 43–67, at pp. 63–5.
5 The study of 'scientific' astrology – theoretical study within
  universities – is distinct from medical astrology, which was much
  more broadly understood and accepted; for more on the differences
  between the two, see Hilary M. Carey, 'Medieval Latin Astrology
  and the Cycles of Life: William English and English Medicine in
  Cambridge, Trinity College MS O.5.26', in *Astro-Medicine*,
  ed. Akasoy, Burnett and Yoeli-Tlalim, pp. 33–54.
6 See Sophie Page, *Astrology in Medieval Manuscripts* (Toronto, 2002);
  and Colum Hourihane, ed., *Time in the Medieval World: Occupations
  of the Months and Signs of the Zodiac in the Index of Christian Art*
  (University Park, PA, 2007).
7 French, 'Astrology in Medical Practice', p. 41.
8 See Isabelle Pantin, 'Analogy and Difference: A Comparative
  Study of Medical and Astronomical Images in Books, 1470–1550',
  in *Observing the World Through Images: Diagrams and Figures in the*

Early-Modern Arts and Sciences, ed. Nicholas Jardine and Isla Fay (Leiden, 2013), pp. 9–44.

9 Harry Bober, 'The Zodiacal Miniature of the *Très Riches Heures* of the Duke of Berry: Its Sources and Meaning', *Journal of the Warburg and Courtauld Institutes*, XI (1948), pp. 1–34.

10 Pedro Gil-Sotres, 'Derivation and Revulsion: The Theory and Practice of Medieval Phlebotomy', in *Practical Medicine*, ed. García-Ballester, French, Arrizabalaga and Cunningham, pp. 110–55, esp. pp. 140–45.

11 Hilary M. Carey, 'What is the Folded Almanac? The Form and Function of a Key Manuscript Source for Astro-Medical Practice in Later Medieval England', *Social History of Medicine*, XVI/3 (2003), pp. 481–509.

12 Adrienne Albright, 'The Heavens on Earth: Practicing and Producing Medieval Astrological Medicine with the Folded Almanac; a Study of Wellcome MS 40', MA diss., Courtauld Institute of Art, 2013.

13 My thanks to Jack Hartnell for bringing this figure to my attention.

14 Alixe Bovey, *Tacuinum Sanitatis: An Early Renaissance Guide to Health* (London, 2005).

15 The moniker *Dreibilderserie* was given to them by Karl Sudhoff, who also named the Five-Figure Series, because of their alleged emergence from German tradition around the same time; see Jack Hartnell, 'Wording the Wound Man', in 'Invention and Imagination in British Art and Architecture, 600–1500', ed. Jessica Berenbeim and Sandy Heslop, special issue, *British Art Studies*, VI (2017), https://doi.org/10.17658/issn.2058-5462/issue-06/jhartnell.

16 There is a non-Western version of a full-figured female body that accompanies Manṣūr ibn Ilyās's *Tashrīḥ-i badan-i insān* (Anatomy of the Human Body), the earliest of which dates to the fifteenth century; see further discussion in Chapter Four.

17 This figure is found in Basel, Universitätsbibliothek, MS D II 11, fol. 170v; see further discussion in Chapter Four.

18 This image is found in the illustrated guide to dissection composed by the surgeon Guido of Vigevano, only preserved in a single manuscript: Chantilly, Bibliothèque du musée Condé, MS 334, fol. 267v; see Chapter Four for further discussion.

19 For more on the Disease Woman, see Katharine Park, *Secrets of Women: Gender, Generation, and the Origins of Human Dissection* (New York, 2010), pp. 106–9; Monica H. Green, *Making Women's Medicine Masculine: The Rise of Male Authority in Pre-Modern*

Gynecology (Oxford, 2008), pp. 153–8; and Tiziana Pesenti,
*Fasciculo de medicina in volgare, Venezia, Giovanni e Gregorio
De Gregori, 1494*, 2 vols (Treviso, 2001), vol. II, pp. 17–18.
20 For more on this idea, see Taylor McCall, 'Functional Abstraction
in Medieval Anatomical Diagrams', in *Abstraction in Medieval Art:
Beyond the Ornament*, ed. Elina Gertsman (Amsterdam, 2021),
pp. 285–308, at pp. 298–300.

3 Cutting Cadavers: Surgeons, Anatomy and the Establishment of Human Dissection

1 As documented by his student, Guy of Chauliac; see Guy de
Chauliac, *Chirurgia magna: Inventarium sive Chirurgia magna
Guigonis de Caulhiaco (Guy de Chauliac)*, ed. Michael R. McVaugh,
2 vols (Leiden, 1997). See also Loren MacKinney, 'The Beginnings
of Western Scientific Anatomy: New Evidence and a Revision
in the Interpretation of Mondeville's Role', *Medical History*, VI/3
(1962), pp. 232–9; and for more on Henry, Marie-Christine
Pouchelle, *The Body and Surgery in the Middle Ages*, trans. Rosemary
Morris (New Brunswick, NJ, 1990).
2 See the copy in London, Royal College of Physicians, MS 227,
fol. 229r (image 467), digitized at http://WDAgo.com, accessed
7 October 2022.
3 Latin transcribed by Julius Leopold Pagel, ed., *Die Anatomie des
Heinrich von Mondeville* (Berlin, 1889), pp. 18–19.
4 Ibid. English translation by Michael McVaugh, 'Surgical Education
in the Middle Ages', *Dynamis: Acta Hispanica ad Medicinae
Scientiarumque Historiam Illustrandam*, XX (2000), pp. 283–304,
at pp. 301–2.
5 Kira Robison has recently re-examined medical teaching at the
University of Bologna between the late thirteenth and early
sixteenth centuries and particularly focused on the establishment of
human dissection and anatomical teaching there. See Kira Robison,
*Healers in the Making: Students, Physicians, and Medical Education
in Medieval Bologna (1250–1550)* (Leiden and Boston, MA, 2021),
esp. chaps. 3 and 4. The foundational study on the establishment
of surgery as a learned discipline is Michael McVaugh, *The Rational
Surgery of the Middle Ages* (Florence, 2006).
6 Robison uses 'extra-curricular' to argue that anatomical texts
indicating the practice existed were being used, but these texts were
not listed as part of the formal curriculum in the 1405 university

statutes (which are the earliest to describe the medical curriculum); *Healers in the Making*, p. 13.

7 For more on the establishment of dissection in Bologna, see Tommaso Duranti, 'Reading the Corpse in the Late Middle Ages (Bologna, Mid-13th Century–Early 16th Century)', in *The Body of Evidence: Corpses and Proofs in Early Modern European Medicine*, ed. Francesco Paolo De Ceglia (Leiden, 2020), pp. 71–104.

8 Michael McVaugh discusses the ways in which medieval surgeons could gain familiarity with the interior spaces of the body other than through human dissection; see Michael McVaugh, 'Fistulas, the Knee, and the "Three-Dimensional" Body', in *Medicine and Space: Body, Surroundings and Borders in Antiquity and the Middle Ages*, ed. Patricia A. Baker, Han Nijdam and Karine van't Land (Leiden and Boston, MA, 2012), pp. 23–36, at pp. 24–7.

9 General works on medieval surgery include McVaugh, *Rational Surgery*; Tony Hunt, *The Medieval Surgery* (Rochester, NY, 1992); and Mirko Grmek, *Mille ans de chirurgie en Occident, ve–xve siècles* (Paris, 1966).

10 Gundolf Keil, 'Roger Frugardi und die Tradition langobardischer Chirurgie', *Sudhoffs Archiv*, LXXXVI (2002), pp. 1–26.

11 Helen Valls, 'Illustrations as Abstracts: The Illustrative Programme in a Montpellier Manuscript of Roger Frugardi's *Chirurgia*', *Medicina nei Secoli*, VIII (1996), pp. 67–83; and Karl Whittington, 'Picturing Christ as Surgeon and Patient in British Library MS Sloane 1977', *Mediaevalia*, XXXV (2014), pp. 83–115.

12 McVaugh, *Rational Surgery*.

13 Danielle Jacquart, *La médecine médiévale dans le cadre parisien: XIVe–XVe siècle* (Paris, 1998), esp. pp. 15–55.

14 Peter Murray Jones, 'John of Arderne and the Mediterranean Tradition of Scholastic Surgery', in *Practical Medicine from Salerno to the Black Death*, ed. Luis García-Ballester, Roger French, Jon Arrizabalaga and Andrew Cunningham (Cambridge, 1994), pp. 298–321.

15 McVaugh, *Rational Surgery*, pp. 32–8.

16 Lanfranc of Milan, *Chirurgia magna* I.2, translated from the Latin in McVaugh, *Rational Surgery*, p. 40, n. 41. McVaugh's source is the 1546 printed edition: Lanfranc, *Ars chirurgica* (Venice, 1546), fol. 209vb.

17 Michael McVaugh, 'When Universities First Encountered Surgery', *Journal of the History of Medicine and Allied Sciences*, LXXII/1 (2017), pp. 6–20.

18 Faith Wallis, ed., *Medieval Medicine: A Reader* (Toronto, 2010), pp. 191–252, for examples of various European university medical curricula.

19 Nancy G. Siraisi, *Taddeo Alderotti and His Pupils: Two Generations of Italian Medical Learning* (Princeton, NJ, 1981).

20 The division of the corpse to bury body parts in different locations gained popularity with the rise of the Crusades, especially among the nobility and royalty. This was evidently a common enough custom to be the subject of a famous condemnatory papal bull issued in 1299, known as the *Detestande feritatis*, or 'abhorred wounds'. Contrary to popular belief, the bull did not specifically forbid human dissection, but it does appear to have slowed the spread of the practice outside Italian universities. For the most comprehensive recent overview, see Immo Warntjes, 'Programmatic Double Burial (Body and Heart) of the European High Nobility, c. 1200–1400: Its Origin, Geography, and Functions', in *Death at Court*, ed. Karl-Heinz Spiess and Immo Warntjes (Wiesbaden, 2012), pp. 197–259. The classic on the subject is Elizabeth A. R. Brown, 'Death and the Human Body in the Later Middle Ages: The Legislation of Boniface VIII on the Division of the Corpse', *Viator*, XII (1981), pp. 221–70.

21 See Katharine Park, 'Masaccio's Skeleton: Art and Anatomy in Renaissance Italy', in *Masaccio's Trinity*, ed. Rona Goffen (Cambridge, 1998), pp. 119–40, at p. 122.

22 George W. Corner published the texts of the Salernitan Demonstrations in *Anatomical Texts of the Earlier Middle Ages: A Study in the Transmission of Culture* (Washington, DC, 1927).

23 Roger French, *Dissection and Vivisection in the European Renaissance* (Aldershot, 1999), pp. 14–15.

24 Katharine Park, *Secrets of Women: Gender, Generation, and the Origins of Human Dissection* (New York, 2006), and Katharine Park, 'The Criminal and the Saintly Body: Autopsy and Dissection in Renaissance Italy', *Renaissance Quarterly*, XLVII/1 (1994), pp. 1–33.

25 Innocent III, *Regestorum sive epistolarum*, liber duodecimus, pontificatus anno XII, christi, 1209, lix, in *Patrologiae cursus completus*, series latina, ed. J. P. Migne, CCXVI (Paris, 1891), cols 64–6. See Ynez Violé O'Neill, 'Innocent III and the Evolution of Anatomy', *Medical History*, XX/4 (1976), pp. 429–33.

26 In Rome, beneath the old Via Latina (now the Via Dino Compagni), is a fourth-century CE fresco depicting an autopsy, or perhaps a dissection, but the exact iconography is debated; see

Curt Proskauer, 'The Significance to Medical History of the Newly Discovered Fourth Century Roman Fresco', *Bulletin of the New York Academy of Medicine*, xxxiv/10 (October 1958), pp. 672–86, and on the frescos in the catacomb more broadly, William Tronzo, *The Via Latina Catacomb: Imitation and Discontinuity in Fourth-Century Roman Painting* (University Park, PA, 1986).

27 Monica H. Green, *The Trotula: A Medieval Compendium of Women's Medicine* (Philadelphia, PA, 2001), pp. 27–30; and Monica H. Green, *Making Women's Medicine Masculine: The Rise of Male Authority in Pre-Modern Gynecology* (Oxford, 2008), pp. 108–9.

28 For an account of alternative interpretations of the iconography of the miniatures, see Taylor McCall, 'Illuminating the Interior: The Illustrations of the Nine Systems of the Body and Anatomical Knowledge in Medieval Europe', PhD diss., University of Cambridge, 2017, pp. 30–32.

29 See Royal Library of the Monastery of San Lorenzo del El Escorial, MS T-I-1, fol. 248r (1280–84, made in Spain), fully digitized here: https://rbdigital.realbiblioteca.es/s/rbme/item/11337, accessed 7 October 2022.. Montserrat Cabré and Fernando Salmón, 'Mining for Poison in a Devout Heart: Dissective Practices and Poisoning in Late Medieval Europe', in *'It All Depends on the Dose': Poisons and Medicines in European History*, ed. Ole Peter Grell, Andrew Cunningham and Jon Arrizabalaga (London, 2018), pp. 43–61. Deirdre Jackson also discusses this song and the connection with other contemporary female autopsies in Deirdre Jackson, 'Saint and Simulacra: Images of the Virgin in the *Cantigas de Santa María* of Alfonso x of Castile (1252–1284)', PhD diss., Courtauld Institute of Art, 2002.

30 Park explores this phenomenon of the autopsies of female religious throughout *Secrets of Women*. For more on Chiara specifically, see Park, 'The Criminal and the Saintly Body', pp. 1–33; and *Secrets of Women*, pp. 39–76.

31 Cabré and Salmón, 'Mining for Poison', pp. 43–4.

32 Duranti, 'Reading the Corpse', pp. 86–9.

33 O'Neill, 'Innocent III', p. 432.

34 Ernest Wickersheimer, *Anatomies de Mondino de Liuzzi et de Guido de Vigevano* (Paris, 1926); and Wallis, ed., *Medieval Medicine: A Reader*, pp. 231–37.

35 Wallis, ed., '47. Academic Dissection as "Material Commentary" (1): Mondino De'Liuzzi', in *Medieval Medicine: A Reader*, p. 232.

36 Ibid., p. 233.

37 Ibid., p. 234.

38 Geneviève Dumas, *Santé et Société à Montpellier à la fin du Moyen Âge* (Leiden and Boston, MA, 2015), pp. 64–5.

39 Wallis, ed., *Medieval Medicine: A Reader*, pp. 203–4.

40 Before the 1470s, there is only one documented human dissection in Germanic lands, which took place at the University of Vienna in 1404. Katharine Park, 'The Life of the Corpse: Dissection and Division in Late Medieval Europe', *Journal of the History of Medicine and Allied Sciences*, L/1 (1995), pp. 111–32, esp. pp. 114–15.

41 Fernando Salmón, 'The Body Inferred: Knowing the Body Through the Dissection of Texts', in *A Cultural History of the Human Body in the Medieval Age*, ed. Linda Kalof (London, 2014), pp. 77–97.

42 Guy de Chauliac, *Chirurgia magna*, ed. McVaugh, vol. I, p. 25.

43 This is the early fourteenth-century London, Royal College of Physicians, MS 227; see n. 2 of this chapter. The two others are Erfurt, Universitätsbibliothek Erfurt, Bibliotheca Amploniana, MS Quart 210, and Berlin, Staatsbibliothek, MS lat. 219. See Taylor McCall, 'Disembodied: Additional MS. 8785 and the Tradition of Human Organ Depictions in Medieval Art and Medicine', *Electronic British Library Journal* (2018), article 8, pp. 1–26, at pp. 21–6, http://vll-minos.bl.uk, accessed 7 October 2022..

44 BnF MS fr. 2030 was catalogued in Alison Stones, *Gothic Manuscripts 1260–1320*, vols II–III of *A Survey of Manuscripts Illuminated in France*, ed. Jonathan J. G. Alexander and François Avril (London and Turnhout, 2013–15), cat. 1–55.

45 *The Western Manuscripts in the Library of Trinity College, Cambridge: A Descriptive Catalogue*, vol. III (Cambridge, 1905), no. O.2.44.

46 For a recent discussion of the emergence and popularity of *memento mori* imagery in both manuscript and sculpture, see Paul Binski, *Gothic Sculpture* (New Haven, CT, 2019), pp. 219–24.

47 Robison discusses the importance of what she calls the 'cadaver survey' (in which physician professors taught their students what a healthy body ought to look like from the cadaver before dissecting) in *Healers in the Making*, pp. 121–3.

48 Lauren Rosenberg, 'Image of Flesh/Flesh of the Image: The Flayed Figure in Henri de Mondeville's *Chirurgia*', *Object*, XX (2019), pp. 82–100.

4 Fourteenth-Century Anatomical Images, Latin West and Islamic Middle East

1 Andreas Vesalius, *The Fabric of the Human Body: An Annotated Translation of the 1543 and 1555 Editions of 'De humani corporis fabrica libri septem'*, trans. and ed. Daniel H. Garrison and Malcolm H. Hast, 2 vols (Basel, 2014). Recent studies on Vesalius that focus on the images in the *Fabrica* include Erika Gielen and Michèle Goyens, eds, *Towards the Authority of Vesalius: Studies on Medicine and the Human Body from Antiquity to the Renaissance and Beyond* (Turnhout, 2018); Rinaldo Canalis and Massimo Ciavolella, eds, *Andreas Vesalius and the 'Fabrica' in the Age of Printing: Art, Anatomy, and Printing in the Italian Renaissance* (Turnhout, 2018); Sachiko Kusukawa, *Picturing the Book of Nature: Image, Text, and Argument in Sixteenth-Century Human Anatomy and Medical Botany* (Chicago, IL, 2012).

2 'To the Divine Charles v, the Mightiest and Most Unvanquished Emperor: Andreas Vesalius' "Preface" to His Books *On the Fabric of the Human Body*', trans. and ed. Daniel H. Garrison and Malcolm H. Hast, online at http://vesalius.northwestern.edu, accessed 1 July 2021.

3 La Bibliothèque virtuelle des manuscrits médiévaux (BVMM) has digitized this manuscript in full: http://bvmm.irht.cnrs.fr/consult/consult.php?reproductionId=16063, accessed 11 January 2019.

4 Guido of Vigevano, *Anatomia Philippi septimi*, Chantilly, Bibliothèque du musée Condé, MS 334, fol. 271r. English translation by Faith Wallis, ed., *Medieval Medicine: A Reader* (Toronto, 2010), pp. 240–41. Regarding the inaccurate perception of a prohibition of dissection by the Church, see n. 20 of Chapter Three.

5 This is 'so that a disease of any member can be recognised, and in what member it is'; Wallis's English translation of the Latin original, *Medieval Medicine: A Reader*, p. 242. This ties in with Kira Robison's idea of the 'cadaver survey' in *Healers in the Making: Students, Physicians, and Medical Education in Medieval Bologna (1250–1550)* (Leiden and Boston, MA, 2021), pp. 121–3.

6 Peter Bovenmyer, 'Dissecting for the King: Guido da Vigevano and the Anatomy of Death', in *Picturing Death, 1200–1600*, ed. Stephen Perkinson and Noa Turel (Leiden, 2019), pp. 213–33.

7 Ernest Wickersheimer, 'L'Anatomie' de Guido de Vigevano, médecin de la reine Jeanne de Bourgogne (1345)', *Archiv für Geschichte der Medizin*, VII (1913), pp. 1–25, at pp. 23–4 (my translation).

8 Katharine Park, 'Masaccio's Skeleton: Art and Anatomy in
   Renaissance Italy', in *Masaccio's Trinity*, ed. Rona Goffen
   (Cambridge, 1998), pp. 119–40, at p. 126. For more on the history
   and iconography of the Three Living and Three Dead, Dance of
   Death, and *transi* tomb skeletons, see Elina Gertsman, *The Dance of
   Death in the Middle Ages: Image, Text, Performance* (Turnhout, 2010),
   esp. the introduction and chap. 1.
9 See Ashby Kinch, 'Image, Ideology, and Form: The Middle
   English Three Dead Kings in Its Iconographic Context', *Chaucer
   Review*, xliii/1 (2008), pp. 49–81.
10 Carole Rawcliffe, 'More than a Bedside Manner: The Political
   Status of the Late Medieval Court Physician', in *St George's Chapel,
   Windsor, in the Late Middle Ages*, ed. C. Richmond and E. Scarff
   (Leeds, 2001), pp. 71–91.
11 Andrew J. Newman, '*Tashrīḥ-i Manṣūr-i*: Human Anatomy Between
   the Galen and Prophetical Medical Traditions', in *La science dans
   le monde iranien à l'époque islamique*, ed. Živa Vesel et al. (Tehran,
   2004), pp. 253–71; and Emilie Savage-Smith, 'Anatomical
   Illustration in Arabic Manuscripts', in *Arab Painting: Text and Image
   in Illustrated Arabic Manuscripts*, ed. Anna Contadini (Leiden,
   2007), pp. 147–59.
12 Savage-Smith details the many types of anatomical images
   in Arabic manuscripts in 'Anatomical Illustration in Arabic
   Manuscripts', and for more on Islamic medicine in general, see
   Peter E. Pormann and Emilie Savage-Smith, *Medieval Islamic
   Medicine* (Edinburgh, 2007).
13 Savage-Smith, 'Anatomical Illustration in Arabic Manuscripts',
   pp. 148–55.
14 By contrast, there are only about a dozen versions of the Western
   Five-Figure Series images.
15 Emilie Savage-Smith, 'Mansur ibn Ilyas, *Tashrih-i badan-i insan*
   (Anatomy of the Human Body)', National Library of Medicine's
   Historical Anatomies on the Web: www.nlm.nih.gov, accessed
   19 April 2021.
16 The manuscript is fully digitized through the University
   of Heidelberg: https://digi.ub.uni-heidelberg.de, accessed
   23 October 2020; see Taylor McCall, 'Illuminating the Interior:
   The Illustrations of the Nine Systems of the Body and Anatomical
   Knowledge in Medieval Europe', PhD diss., University of Cambridge,
   2017, pp. 115–31; and Karl Sudhoff, *Ein Beitrag zur Geschichte
   der Anatomie im Mittelalter speziell der anatomischen Graphik nach*

Handschriften des 9. bis 15. Jahrhunderts (Leipzig, 1908; repr. Hildesheim, 1964), pp. 11–51.

17 Savage-Smith, 'Anatomical Illustration in Arabic Manuscripts', p. 158.

18 Roger French, 'An Origin for the Bone Text of the "Five-Figure Series"', *Sudhoffs Archiv*, 68 (1984), pp. 143–58.

19 These are Aristotle's *Metaphysica* with commentary by Augustine of Ancona, Aristotle's *Physica*, and an anonymous tripartite treatise on logic, ethics and physics; see McCall, 'Illuminating the Interior', pp. 121–3.

20 McCall, 'Illuminating the Interior', pp. 123–7.

21 The accompanying anatomical images in the Basel and Vatican manuscripts (the Munich manuscript has no other drawings) are very different; the Basel drawings are carefully rendered illustrations, large and uncluttered, while the Vatican drawings are unfinished sketches, difficult to conclusively identify, clustered together with other medical drawings on damaged parchment.

22 Alison Stones, *Gothic Manuscripts, 1260–1320*, vols II–III of *A Survey of Manuscripts Illuminated in France*, ed. Jonathan J. G. Alexander and François Avril (London and Turnhout, 2013–15), cat. VII–6.

23 Michael Camille, 'Image and the Self: Unwriting Later Medieval Bodies', in *Framing Medieval Bodies*, ed. Sarah Kay and Miri Rubin (Manchester, 1994), pp. 62–100, at pp. 82–3.

5 Decorating the Text: Professional Artists and the Anatomical Page

1 While the focus here is on miniatures and other illuminations, the standard work on the division and layout of scholastic texts is M. B. Parkes, 'The Influence of the Concepts of *Ordinatio* and *Compilatio* on the Development of the Book', in *Scribes, Scripts, and Readers: Studies in the Communication, Presentation, and Dissemination of Medieval Texts* (London, 1991), pp. 35–70.

2 Anne D. Hedeman, 'Gothic Manuscript Illustration: The Case of France', in *A Companion to Medieval Art: Romanesque and Gothic in Northern Europe*, ed. Conrad Rudolph (Oxford, 2006), pp. 421–42; Richard H. Rouse and Mary A. Rouse, *Manuscripts and Their Makers: Commercial Book Producers in Medieval Paris, 1200–1500* (Turnhout, 1999); and Robert Branner, *Manuscript Painting in Paris during the Reign of St. Louis* (Berkeley, CA, 1977).

3 Vern L. Bullough, 'The Medieval Medical University at Paris',
   Bulletin of the History of Medicine, XXXI (1957), pp. 197–211.
4 This is known as the pecia system. See the seminal Jean A. Destrez,
   La pecia dans les manuscrits universitaires du XIIIe et du XIVe siècle
   (Paris, 1935); Graham Pollard, 'The Pecia System in the Medieval
   Universities', in *Medieval Scribes, Manuscripts and Libraries:
   Essays Presented to N.R. Ker*, ed. M. B. Parkes and Andrew G.
   Watson (London, 1978), pp. 145–61; and more recently Nikolaus
   Weichselbaumer, '"Quod Exemplaria vera habeant et correcta":
   Concerning the Distribution and Purpose of the Pecia System',
   in *Specialist Markets in the Early Modern Book World*, ed. Richard
   Kirwan and Sophie Mullins (Leiden and Boston, MA, 2015),
   pp. 331–50.
5 A recent work tackling the encyclopaedic tradition is Mary
   Franklin-Brown, *Reading the World: Encyclopedic Writing in the
   Scholastic Age* (Chicago, IL, 2012).
6 See especially Angela Montford, *Health, Sickness, Medicine and the
   Friars in the Thirteenth and Fourteenth Centuries* (Aldershot, 2004).
7 Mary Niven Alston, 'The Attitude of the Church Towards
   Dissection Before 1500', *Bulletin of the History of Medicine*, XVI/3
   (1944), pp. 221–38.
8 For a discussion of the incorporation of Galenic anatomy in
   medieval works, see R. K. French, '*De Juvamentis Membrorum* and
   the Reception of Galenic Physiological Anatomy', *Isis*, LXX (1979),
   pp. 96–109.
9 See Nancy G. Siraisi, *Avicenna in Renaissance Italy: The 'Canon'
   and Medical Teaching in Italian Universities after 1500* (Princeton, NJ,
   1987), esp. 'The *Canon* of Avicenna', pp. 19–40; and 'The *Canon* in
   the Medieval Universities and the Humanist Attack on Avicenna',
   pp. 43–76.
10 Luke Demaitre, *Medieval Medicine: The Art of Healing, from Head
   to Toe* (Santa Barbara, CA, 2013).
11 For general information about *De proprietatibus rerum* and
   Bartholomew, see Elizabeth Keen, *The Journey of a Book:
   Bartholomew the Englishman and the Properties of Things* (Canberra,
   2007); J. G. Lidaka and P. Binkley, 'Bartholomaeus Anglicus in
   the Thirteenth Century', *Brill's Studies in Intellectual History*, LXXIX
   (1997), pp. 393–406; and M. C. Seymour, *Bartholomaeus Anglicus
   and His Encyclopaedia* (Aldershot, 1992).
12 Taylor McCall, 'Disembodied: Additional MS. 8785 and the
   Tradition of Human Organ Depictions in Medieval Art and

Medicine', *Electronic British Library Journal* (2018), article 8,
pp. 1–26, available http://vll-minos.bl.uk, accessed 7 October 2022.

13 See Alison Stones, *Gothic Manuscripts, 1260–1320*, vols II–III
of *A Survey of Manuscripts Illuminated in France*, ed. Jonathan
J. G. Alexander and François Avril (London and Turnhout,
2013–15), cat. 1–58; Amandine Postec, 'Un exemplaire singulier
du *De animalibus* d'Albert le Grand et son illustration (Paris, BnF,
Manuscrits, Latin 16169)', *Reinardus: Yearbook of the International
Reynard Society*, XXVI (2014), pp. 137–60; and Jack Hartnell,
'The Body Inside-Out: Anatomical Memory at Maubuisson Abbey',
Art History, XLII/2 (2019), pp. 242–73.

14 Kenneth Kitchell Jr and Irven Michael Resnick, trans. and eds,
Albertus Magnus 'On Animals': A Medieval 'Summa Zoologica',
2 vols (Baltimore, MD, 1999).

15 See Branner's description of the workshop in *Manuscript Painting*,
pp. 82–6, and his earlier article, 'The Johannes Grusch Atelier
and the Continental Origins of the William of Devon Painter',
Art Bulletin, LIV (1972), pp. 24–30.

16 Angela Montford, '"Brothers who have Studied Medicine":
Dominican Friars in Thirteenth-Century Paris', *Social History of
Medicine*, XXIV/3 (2011), pp. 535–55, at p. 547. There are a number
of issues in attempting to assign a style to a particular workshop,
a subject that will not be delved into too deeply here.

17 Stones, *Gothic Manuscripts*, cat. 1–8.

18 Montford, '"Brothers"', pp. 537–55.

19 Ibid., pp. 542–44.

20 However, there is an account of a post-mortem examination
taking place there in 1407, on the body of the Bishop of Arras,
to determine how he had died in order to be able to treat others
suffering from a similar disease; see Bullough, 'The Medieval
Medical University at Paris', p. 210.

21 Stones, *Gothic Manuscripts, 1260–1320*, cat. 1–8; see also Monica H.
Green, 'Richard de Fournival and the Reconfiguration of Learned
Medicine in the 13th Century', in *Richard de Fournival et les sciences
au XIIIe siècle*, ed. Joëlle Ducos and Christopher Lucken (Florence,
2018), pp. 179–206, at pp. 203–6.

22 Loren C. MacKinney, 'Medical Illustrations in Medieval
Manuscripts of the Vatican Library (concluded)', *Manuscripta*, 3
(1959), pp. 76–88; for more bibliography and the fully digitized
manuscripts, see the Biblioteca Apostolica digitized manuscripts
website: https://digi.vatlib.it/mss, accessed 30 October 2021.

23 'De Arte Phisicali et de Chirurgia' by John Arderne; From a New Digital
   Version of the Stockholm Roll, trans. and commentary by Torgny
   Svenberg and Peter Murray Jones (Stockholm, 2014).

24 Faith Wallis has recently explored the potential 'use' of the
   Stockholm Roll, particularly as pertains to the foetal images in
   relation to Philippa of England: Faith Wallis, 'Between Reading
   and Doing: The Case of Medieval Manuscript Books of Practical
   Medicine', in The Edinburgh History of Reading: Early Readers,
   ed. Mary Hammond (Edinburgh, 2020), pp. 115–34, esp.
   pp. 118–19 and 127–9.

25 For more on Arderne's treatment of noblemen, see Marion Turner,
   'Thomas Usk and John Arderne', Chaucer Review, XLVII/1 (2012),
   pp. 95–105.

26 Peter Murray Jones, '"Sicut hic depingitur . . .": John of Arderne
   and English Medical Illustration in the 14th and 15th Centuries',
   in Die Kunst und das Studium der Natur vom 14. zum 16. Jahrhundert,
   ed. Wolfram Prinz and Andreas Beyer (Berlin, 1987), pp. 103–26;
   and Peter Murray Jones, 'Staying with the Programme: Illustrated
   Manuscripts of John of Arderne, c. 1380–c. 1550', in Decoration
   and Illustration in Medieval English Manuscripts, English Manuscript
   Studies, 1100–1700, vol. X, ed. A.S.G. Edwards (London, 2002),
   pp. 204–27.

27 Peter Murray Jones has traced the reception of Italian and other
   southern European scholastic surgical manuals in England and
   specifically in Arderne's writings in Peter Murray Jones, 'John of
   Arderne and the Mediterranean Tradition of Scholastic Surgery',
   in Practical Medicine from Salerno to the Black Death, ed. Luis García-
   Ballester, Roger French, Jon Arrizabalaga and Andrew Cunningham
   (Cambridge, 1994), pp. 289–321.

28 See especially Michael Camille's work on marginal imagery, for
   example, Image on the Edge: The Margins of Medieval Art (London,
   1992).

29 S.A.J. Moorat, Catalogue of Western Manuscripts on Medicine and
   Science in the Wellcome Historical Medical Library (London,
   1962–73), no. 290; and for information on the images, see Kathleen
   L. Scott, Later Gothic Manuscripts, 1390–1490, 2 vols, in A Survey of
   Manuscripts Illuminated in the British Isles, 5 (London, 1996), vol. I,
   pl. 106–7; vol. II, no. 99, 275–7.

30 For more on the texts, see Linda Ehrsam Voigts and Patricia Deery
   Kurtz, Scientific and Medical Writings in Old and Middle English, nos
   4608 and 1873, available online at https://cctr1.umkc.edu, accessed

21 October 2022; and Jesús Romero-Barranco, *The Late Middle English Version of Constantinus Africanus' 'Venerabilis Anatomia' in London, Wellcome Library, MS 290 (ff. 1r–41v)* (Newcastle-upon-Tyne, 2015).

31 Tiziana Pesenti, *Fasciculo de medicina in volgare, Venezia, Giovanni e Gregorio De Gregori, 1494*, 2 vols (Treviso, 2001), vol. II, pp. 1–42; and Jack Hartnell, 'Wording the Wound Man', in Jessica Berenbeim and Sandy Heslop, eds, 'Invention and Imagination in British Art and Architecture, 600–1500', special issue, *British Art Studies*, VI (2017), https://doi.org/10.17658/issn.2058-5462/issue-06/jhartnell.

32 Katharine Park, 'Masaccio's Skeleton: Art and Anatomy in Renaissance Italy', in *Masaccio's Trinity*, ed. Rona Goffen (Cambridge, 1998), pp. 119–40, at pp. 121–2.

33 Lorenzo Ghiberti, *I commentarii (Biblioteca Nazionale Centrale di Firenze, II, I, 333)*, ed. Lorenzo Bartoli (Florence, 1998), II.10, p. 50 (my translation).

34 Literature on the Renaissance turn to naturalism, as well as cautions against over-reliance on the idea, is extensive; the most recent and helpful to this study were Jean A. Givens, *Observation and Image-Making in Gothic Art* (Cambridge, 2005); Vivian Nutton, 'Representation and Memory in Renaissance Anatomical Illustration', in *Immagini per Conoscere: Dal Rinascimento alla Rivoluzione scientifica. Atti della Giornata di Studio (Firenze, Palazzo Strozzi, 29 ottobre 1999)*, ed. Fabrizio Meroi and Claudio Pogliano (Florence, 2001), pp. 61–80; and Martin Kemp, 'Taking it on Trust: Form and Meaning in Naturalistic Representation', *Archives of Natural History*, XVII/2 (1990), pp. 127–88.

35 Bernard Schultz, *Art and Anatomy in Renaissance Italy* (Ann Arbor, MI, 1985), pp. 2–3; and Park, 'Masaccio's Skeleton', pp. 119–21.

36 Park, 'Masaccio's Skeleton', pp. 128–33.

37 Schultz, *Art and Anatomy*, pp. 3–4.

38 The bibliography on Leonardo and his anatomical explorations is extensive. Particularly useful for this study were Martin Kemp, *Leonardo da Vinci: Experience, Experiment and Design* (London, 2006), pp. 257–61 and 285–94; Domenico Laurenza, *Art and Anatomy in Renaissance Italy: Images from a Scientific Revolution*, trans. Frank Dabell (New York and New Haven, CT, 2012), pp. 10–13; and Schultz, *Art and Anatomy*, pp. 67–100.

39 For a recent assessment of Leonardo's unrealistic takes on human anatomy, see Alessandro Nova, '"La Dolce Morte". Die anatomischen Zeichnungen Leonardo da Vincis als

Erkenntnismittel und reflektierte Kunstpraxis', in *Zergliederungen: Anatomie und Wahrnehmung in der Frühen Neuzeit*, ed. Albert Schirrmeister and Mathias Pozsgai (Frankfurt, 2005), pp. 136–63.

40 Laurenza, *Art and Anatomy in Renaissance Italy*, pp. 13–20.

41 Jacopo Berengario da Carpi, *A Short Introduction to Anatomy (Isagogae breves)*, trans. L. R. Lind (Chicago, IL, 1959).

42 Laurenza, *Art and Anatomy in Renaissance Italy*, p. 19.

43 Roger French, 'Berengario da Carpi and the Use of Commentary in Anatomical Teaching', in *The Medical Renaissance of the Sixteenth Century*, ed. Andrew Wear et al. (Cambridge, 1985), pp. 42–74, at pp. 61–2.

44 For more on counterfeit printing of anatomical scenes, see Sachiko Kusukawa, *Picturing the Book of Nature: Image, Text, and Argument in Sixteenth-Century Human Anatomy and Medical Botany* (Chicago, IL, 2012), pp. 8–12.

45 Vincent Mayr, 'Hagenauer [von Hagnow; Hagnower], Nikolaus', *Grove Art Online* (2003), www.oxfordartonline.com, accessed 13 December 2020.

6 The Anatomy of a Scene: Dissection in Manuscript and Print, *c.* 1400–1540

1 Nancy G. Siraisi, *Medieval and Early Renaissance Medicine: An Introduction to Knowledge and Practice* (Chicago, IL, 1990); and Luis Garcia-Ballester, Roger French, Jon Arrizabalaga and Andrew Cunningham, eds, *Practical Medicine from Salerno to the Black Death* (Cambridge, 1994).

2 See, for instance, the popular *Tacuinum sanitatis* (Maintenance of Health); Alixe Bovey, *Tacuinum Sanitatis: An Early Renaissance Guide to Health* (London, 2005).

3 For more on early printed medical images, see Peter Murray Jones, 'Visualization in Medicine between Script and Print, *c.* 1375–1550', in *The Visualization of Knowledge in Medieval and Early Modern Europe*, ed. Marica Kupfer, Adam S. Cohen and J. H. Chajes (Turnhout, 2020), pp. 341–60.

4 Portions of this chapter appeared in print in Taylor McCall, 'Anatomical Icon: Dissection Scenes in Manuscript and Print, *c.* 1350–1540', in 'Anatomical Things', special issue, *KNOW: Journal for the History of Knowledge*, x (2022), pp. 7–46.

5 Andreas Vesalius, *The Fabric of the Human Body: An Annotated Translation of the 1543 and 1555 Editions of 'De humani corporis*

fabrica libri septem', trans. and ed. Daniel H. Garrison and Malcolm H. Hast, 2 vols (Basel, 2014). Recent studies on Vesalius that focus on the images in the *Fabrica* include Erika Gielen and Michèle Goyens, eds, *Towards the Authority of Vesalius: Studies on Medicine and the Human Body from Antiquity to the Renaissance and Beyond* (Turnhout, 2018); Rinaldo Canalis and Massimo Ciavolella, eds, *Andreas Vesalius and the 'Fabrica' in the Age of Printing: Art, Anatomy, and Printing in the Italian Renaissance* (Turnhout, 2018); and Sachiko Kusukawa, *Picturing the Book of Nature: Image, Text, and Argument in Sixteenth-Century Human Anatomy and Medical Botany* (Chicago, IL, 2012).

6 See Katharine Park, *Secrets of Women: Gender, Generation, and the Origins of Human Dissection* (New York, 2006), especially pp. 207–59, for more on the female corpse in the frontispiece.

7 BnF MS fr. 218, fol. 401v. See Paulin Paris, *Les manuscrits françois de la bibliothèque du roi leur histoire et celle des textes allemands anglois hollandois italiens espagnols de la même collection*, vol. II (Paris, 1836), no. 223, pp. 220–21; and Marie-José Imbault-Huart, ed., *La médecine au Moyen Âge à travers les manuscrits de la Bibliothèque nationale* (Paris, 1983), no. 41, pp. 106–7.

8 Bartholomew the Englishman, *Livre des proprietés des choses*, trans. Jean Corbichon, ed. Pierre Farget, printed by Johannes Siber (Lyon, c. 1484–6), ISTC no. ibo0143800.

9 'Dictionnaire des imprimeurs et libraires lyonnais du quinzième siècle', *Revue française d'histoire du livre*, 118–21 (2003), pp. 209–64, no. 137, pp. 253–4.

10 Bibliography on this subject is extensive; for recent works with further sources, see Sonja Drimmer, ed., *Manual Impressions: Visualizing Print in Manuscript, Europe, circa 1450–circa 1850*, special issue of *Digital Philology: A Journal of Medieval Cultures*, IX (2020), especially Drimmer's 'Introduction: The Manuscript Copy and the Printed Original in the Digital Present', pp. 93–119; Cristina Dondi, ed., *Printing R-Evolution and Society 1450–1500: Fifty Years that Changed Europe*, Studi di storia, XIII (2020), doi:10.30687/978-88-6969-332-8; and Lotte Hellinga, *Texts in Transit: Manuscript to Proof and Print in the Fifteenth Century* (Leiden, 2014).

11 Bartholomew the Englishman, *Livre des proprietés des choses*.

12 'Dictionnaire des imprimeurs', pp. 237, 254.

13 For more on the cost of incunabula, see Neil Harris, 'Costs We Don't Think About: An Unusual Copy of Franciscus de Platea,

Opus restitutionum (1474), and a Few Other Items', in *Printing R-Evolution and Society*, ed. Dondi, pp. 511–40.

14 On anatomies as 'civic events' see Park, *Secrets of Women*, esp. p. 88; and Katharine Park, 'The Criminal and the Saintly Body: Autopsy and Dissection in Renaissance Italy', *Renaissance Quarterly*, XLVII/1 (1994), pp. 1–33.

15 Mireille Vial, '*Scriptor et medicus*: la médecine dans les manuscrits de la Bibliothèque interuniversitaire de Montpellier', electronic resource (Montpellier, 2011), https://manuscrits.biu-montpellier.fr, accessed 9 May 2020.

16 Charles Singer, 'A Study in Early Renaissance Anatomy, with a New Text: The *Anothomia* of Hieronymo Manfredi, Transcribed and Translated by A. Mildred Westland', in *Studies in the History and Method of Science*, ed. Charles Singer (Oxford, 1917), pp. 79–164.

17 These images have not benefitted from much study. A full catalogue description and bibliography can be found on the University of Glasgow's website: http://collections.gla.ac.uk, accessed 18 June 2020. The only identifying information in this manuscript is the shield of the Order of the Golden Fleece, a chivalric order of knighthood founded by Philip III, Duke of Burgundy ('Philip the Good'), in 1429.

18 See Andrea Carlino, *Books of the Body: Anatomical Ritual and Renaissance Learning*, trans. John Tedeschi and Anne C. Tedeschi (Chicago, IL, 1999), pp. 33–8.

19 Mundinus, *Anatomia*, ed. Martinus Polichius de Mellerstadt, printed by Martin Landsberg (Leipzig, c. 1493), ISTC no. im00874000.

20 See Tiziana Pesenti, *Fasciculo de medicina in volgare, Venezia, Giovanni e Gregorio De Gregori, 1494*, 2 vols (Treviso, 2001); Chris Coppens, *De vele levens van een boek: de Fasciculus medicinae opnieuw bekeken* (Brussels, 2009); and the recent online exhibition by the New York Academy of Medicine, which has examples from many of the editions, with essays by Taylor McCall and Natalie Lussey Seale: '*Facendo il Libro*: The Making of *Fasciculus Medicinae*, an Early Printed Anatomy' (2018), http://digitalcollections.nyam.org, accessed 1 July 2021.

21 See Pesenti, *Fasciculo di medicina in volgare*, vol. II, pp. 49–51; and Chris Coppens, '"For the Benefit of Ordinary People": The Dutch Translation of the *Fasciculus medicinae*, Antwerp 1512', *Quaerendo*, XXXIX (2009), pp. 168–205, at pp. 169–71.

22 The sixth image, a urine wheel, was also a common manuscript diagram, consulted by physicians to help diagnose patients based on the colour, smell and taste of their urine.

23 The Italian edition was translated by Sebastiano Manilio and again printed by the Gregori brothers in Venice; see Pesenti, *Fasciculo de medicina in volgare*, and Tiziana Pesenti, 'Editoria medica tra Quattro e Cinquecento: l' "Articella" e il "*Fasciculus medicine*"', in *Trattati scientifici nel Veneto fra il xv e xvi ssecolo*, ed. Ezio Riondato (Venice, 1985), pp. 1–28.

24 Jerome J. Bylebyl, 'Interpreting the *Fasciculo* Anatomy Scene', *Journal of the History of Medicine and Allied Sciences*, xlv/3 (1990), pp. 285–316.

25 Monique Kornell, 'Jan Steven van Calcar, *c*. 1515–*c*. 1546, Vesalius's Illustrator', in *Andreas Vesalius and the 'Fabrica'*, ed. Canalis and Ciavolella, pp. 99–130; Michelangelo Muraro, 'Tiziano e le Anatomie del Vesalio', in *Tiziano e Venezia: Convegno internazionale di studi, Venezia* (Vicenza, 1980), pp. 307–16; and Martin Kemp, 'A Drawing for the *Fabrica* and Some Thoughts upon the Vesalius Muscle-Men', *Medical History*, xiv (1970), pp. 277–88.

26 Translation by Faith Wallis, ed., '47. Academic Dissection as "Material Commentary" (1): Mondino De'Liuzzi', in *Medieval Medicine: A Reader* (Toronto, 2010), p. 232.

SELECT BIBLIOGRAPHY

Belloni, Luigi, 'Gli schemi anatomici trecenteschi (serie dei cinque
    sistemi e occhio) del codice trivulziano 836', *Rivista di Storia delle
    Scienze Mediche e Naturali*, XLI (1950), pp. 193–212
Brown, Elizabeth A. R., 'Death and the Human Body in the Later
    Middle Ages: The Legislation of Boniface VIII on the Division of
    the Corpse', *Viator*, XII (1981), pp. 221–70
Bylebyl, Jerome J., 'Interpreting the *Fasciculo* Anatomy Scene',
    Journal of the History of Medicine and Allied Sciences, XLV/3 (1990),
    pp. 285–316
Cadden, Joan, *Meanings of Sex Difference in the Middle Ages: Medicine,
    Science, and Culture* (Cambridge, 1993, 1995)
Camille, Michael, 'Before the Gaze: The Internal Senses and Late
    Medieval Practices of Seeing', in *Visuality Before and Beyond
    the Renaissance*, ed. Robert S. Nelson (Cambridge, 2000),
    pp. 197–223
Carlino, Andrea, *Books of the Body: Anatomical Ritual and Renaissance
    Learning*, trans. John Tedeschi and Anne C. Tedeschi (Chicago, IL,
    1999)
—, *Paper Bodies: A Catalogue of Anatomical Fugitive Sheets, 1538–1687*,
    trans. Noga Arikha (London, 1999)
Carruthers, Mary, *The Book of Memory: A Study of Memory in Medieval
    Culture* (Cambridge, 2008)
Choulant, Ludwig, *History and Bibliography of Anatomic Illustration*,
    trans. Mortimer Frank (Chicago, IL, 1920)
Cohen, Adam S., 'Making Memories in a Medieval Miscellany', *Gesta*,
    XLVIII (2009), special issue: *Making Thoughts, Making Pictures,
    Making Memories in Late Antiquity and the Middle Ages: Essays in
    Honor of Mary Carruthers*, ed. Anne D. Hedeman, pp. 135–52
Coppens, Chris, *De vele levens van een boek: de Fasciculus medicinae
    opnieuw bekeken* (Brussels, 2009)
Corner, George W., *Anatomical Texts of the Earlier Middle Ages:
    A Study in the Transmission of Culture* (Washington, DC, 1927)
Cunningham, Andrew, *The Anatomical Renaissance* (Aldershot, 1997)
De Ceglia, Francesco Paolo, ed., *The Body of Evidence: Corpses and
    Proofs in Early Modern European Medicine* (Leiden, 2020)

Drimmer, Sonja, ed., *Digital Philology: A Journal of Medieval Cultures*,
    IX (2020) special issue: *Manual Impressions: Visualizing Print in
    Manuscript, Europe, circa 1450–circa 1850*

Edelstein, Ludwig, 'The History of Anatomy in Antiquity', in *Ancient
    Medicine: Selected Papers of Ludwig Edelstein*, ed. Owsei Temkin and
    C. Lilian Temkin (Baltimore, MD, 1967), pp. 247–301

Evans, Michael, 'The Geometry of the Mind: Scientific Diagrams and
    Medieval Thought', *Architectural Association Quarterly*, XII (1980),
    pp. 32–55

Ferckel, Christoph, 'Diagramme der sexualorgane in mittelalterliche
    Handschriften', *Archiv für Geschichte der Medizin*, X (1917),
    pp. 255–63

Fowler, Alastair, *Renaissance Realism: Narrative Images in Literature
    and Art* (Oxford, 2003)

French, Roger, 'Berengario da Carpi and the Use of Commentary in
    Anatomical Teaching', in *The Medical Renaissance of the Sixteenth
    Century*, ed. Andrew Wear et al. (Cambridge, 1985), pp. 42–74

—, *Dissection and Vivisection in the European Renaissance* (Aldershot,
    1999)

—, 'A Note on the Anatomical Accessus of the Middle Ages', *Medical
    History*, XXIII (1979), pp. 461–8

Garcia-Ballester, Luis, Roger French, Jon Arrizabalaga and Andrew
    Cunningham, eds, *Practical Medicine from Salerno to the Black Death*
    (Cambridge, 1994)

Givens, Jean A., Karen M. Reeds and Alain Touwaide, eds, *Visualising
    Medieval Medicine and Natural History, 1200–1550* (Aldershot,
    2006)

Green, Monica H., 'From "Diseases of Women" to "Secrets of Women":
    The Transformation of Gynecological Literature in the Later
    Middle Ages', *Journal of Medieval and Early Modern Studies*, XXX/1
    (2000), pp. 5–40

—, '"Habeo istos libros phisicales": The Changing Form, Content, and
    Professional Function of the Medical Book in the Long Twelfth
    Century', in *The European Book in the Long Twelfth Century*,
    ed. Erik Kwakkel and Rodney Thomson (Cambridge, 2019)

—, *Making Women's Medicine Masculine: The Rise of Male Authority
    in Pre-Modern Gynecology* (Oxford, 2008)

Hartnell, Jack, 'Wording the Wound Man', *British Art Studies*, special
    issue: 'Medieval Invention and Imagination' (2017)

Herrlinger, Robert, *History of Medical Illustration from Antiquity
    to AD 1600* (Nijkerk, 1970)

Hill, Boyd H., Jr, 'Another Member of the Sudhoff *Fünfbilderserie* – Wellcome MS 5000', *Sudhoffs Archiv für Geschichte der Medizin und der Naturwissenchaften*, XLIII (1959), pp. 13–19

—, 'The *Fünfbilderserie* and Medieval Anatomy', PhD diss., University of North Carolina (1963)

—, 'The Grain and the Spirit in Medieval Anatomy', *Speculum*, XL (1965), pp. 63–73

—, 'A Medieval German Wound Man: Wellcome MS 49', *Journal of the History of Medicine and Allied Sciences*, XX (1965), pp. 334–57

Jacquart, Danielle, 'The Influence of Arabic Medicine in the West', in *Encyclopaedia of the History of Arabic Science*, ed. Roshdi Rashed and Régis Morelon (London, 1996), pp. 917–38

—, and Francoise Micheau, *La médecine arabe et l'occident médiéval* (Paris, 1990)

Jones, Peter Murray, *Medieval Medicine in Illuminated Manuscripts* (London, 1998)

—, '"Sicut hic depingitur . . .": John of Arderne and English Medical Illustration in the 14th and 15th Centuries', in *Die Kunst und das Studium der Natur vom 14. zum 16. Jahrhundert*, ed. Wolfram Prinz and Andreas Beyer (Berlin, 1987), pp. 103–26

Kay, Sarah, and Miri Rubin, eds, *Framing Medieval Bodies* (Manchester, 1994)

Klemm, Tanja, *Bildphysiologie: Wahrnehmung und Körper in Mittelalter und Renaissance* (Berlin, 2010)

Kurz, Otto, 'The Medical Illustrations of the Wellcome MS', *Journal of the Warburg and Courtauld Institutes*, V, Appendix 2 (1942), pp. 137–42

Kusukawa, Sachiko, *Picturing the Book of Nature: Image, Text, and Argument in Sixteenth-Century Human Anatomy and Medical Botany* (Chicago, IL, 2012)

Laurenza, Domenico, *Art and Anatomy in Renaissance Italy: Images from a Scientific Revolution*, trans. Frank Dabell (New York and New Haven, CT, 2012)

McCall, Taylor, 'Anatomical Icon: Dissection Scenes in Manuscript and Print, *c.* 1350–1540', *KNOW: Journal for the History of Knowledge*, Special Issue: 'Anatomical Things', X (2022), pp. 7–46

—, 'Disembodied: Additional MS. 8785 and the Tradition of Human Organ Depictions in Medieval Art and Medicine', *Electronic British Library Journal* (2018), article 8, pp. 1–26, http://vll-minos.bl.uk, accessed 7 October 2022

—, 'Functional Abstraction in Medieval Anatomical Diagrams',
    in *Abstraction in Medieval Art: Beyond the Ornament*, ed. Elina
    Gertsman (Amsterdam, 2021), pp. 285–308

—, 'Illuminating the Interior: The Illustrations of the Nine Systems
    of the Body and Anatomical Knowledge in Medieval Europe',
    PhD diss., University of Cambridge, 2017

—, '*Reliquam dicit pictura*: Text and Image in an Illustrated Anatomical
    Manual (Gonville and Caius College, MS 190/223)', *Transactions of
    the Cambridge Bibliographical Society*, XVI (2016), pp. 1–22

Maccagni, Carlo, 'Frammento di un codice di medicina del secolo XIV
    (manoscritto N. 735. già codice Roncioni N. 99) della Biblioteca
    Universitaria di Pisa', *Physis*, XI (1969), pp. 311–78

MacKinney, Loren, 'Beginnings of Western Scientific Anatomy: New
    Evidence and A Revision in Interpretation of Mondeville's Role',
    Medical History, VI (1960), pp. 233–9

—, and Harry Bober, 'A Thirteenth-Century Medical Case History
    in Miniatures', *Speculum*, XXXV (1960), pp. 251–9

—, and Boyd H. Hill Jr, 'A New *Fünfbilderserie* Manuscript – Vatican
    Palat. Lat. 1110', *Sudhoffs Archiv für Geschichte der Medizin und
    der Naturwissenchaften*, XLVIII (1964), pp. 323–30

—, and Thomas Herndon, *Medical Illustrations in Medieval Manuscripts*
    (London, 1965)

McVaugh, Michael, ed., *Chirurgia magna: Inventarium sive Chirurgia
    magna Guigonis de Caulhiaco (Guy de Chauliac)*, 2 vols (Leiden,
    1997)

—, trans., 'Guy de Chauliac, History of Surgery', in *A Source Book
    in Medieval Science*, ed. Edward Grant (Cambridge, MA, 1974)

—, *The Rational Surgery of the Middle Ages* (Florence, 2006)

Marchetti, Francesca, 'Educating the Midwife: The Role of Illustrations
    in Late Antique and Medieval Obstetrical Texts', in *Pregnancy
    and Childbirth in the Premodern World: European and Middle Eastern
    Cultures, from Late Antiquity to the Renaissance*, ed. Costanza Gislon
    Dopfel, Alessandra Foscati and Charles Burnett (Turnhout, 2019),
    pp. 3–28

Murdoch, John E., *Album of Science: Antiquity and the Middle Ages*
    (New York, 1984)

Newman, Andrew J., 'Tashrīḥ-i Manṣūr-i: Human Anatomy Between
    the Galen and Prophetical Medical Traditions', in *La science
    dans le monde iranien à l'époque islamique*, ed. Živa Vesel, Hossein
    Beikbaghban and Bertrand Thierry de Crussol Des Épesse [1998]
    (Tehran, 2004), pp. 253–71

Nutton, Vivian, 'Representation and Memory in Renaissance
    Anatomical Illustration', in *Immagini per Conoscere: Dal
    Rinascimento alla Rivoluzione scientifica. Atti della Giornata di Studio
    (Firenze, Palazzo Strozzi, 29 ottobre 1999)*, ed. Fabrizio Meroi and
    Claudio Pogliano (Florence, 2001), pp. 61–80
O'Neill, Ynez Violé, 'Diagrams of the Medieval Brain', in *Iconography
    at the Crossroads, Index of Christian Art*, ed. Brendan Cassidy
    (Princeton, NJ, 1990), pp. 91–105
——, 'The *Fünfbilderserie* – a Bridge to the Unknown', *Bulletin of the
    History of Medicine*, LI (1977), pp. 538–49
——, 'The *Fünfbilderserie* Reconsidered', *Bulletin of the History of Medicine*,
    XLIII (1969), pp. 236–45
——, 'Innocent III and the Evolution of Anatomy', *Medical History*, XX
    (1976), pp. 429–33
——, 'Meningeal Localization: A New Key to Some Medical Texts,
    Diagrams and Practices of the Middle Ages', *Mediaevistik*, VI (1993),
    pp. 211–38
——, 'Tracing Islamic Influences in an Illustrated Anatomical Manual',
    Bulletin of Islamic Medicine, II (1982), pp. 154–62
Park, Katharine, 'The Criminal and the Saintly Body: Autopsy and
    Dissection in Renaissance Italy', *Renaissance Quarterly*, XLVII/I
    (1994), pp. 1–33
——, 'Masaccio's Skeleton: Art and Anatomy in Renaissance Italy', in
    Masaccio's Trinity, ed. Rona Goffen (Cambridge, 1998), pp. 119–40
——, *Secrets of Women: Gender, Generation, and the Origins of Human
    Dissection* (New York, 2006)
Pesenti, Tiziana, 'Editoria medica tra Quattro e Cinquecento: l'
    "Articella" e il "Fasciculus medicine"', in *Trattati scientifici nel Veneto
    fra il XV e XVI secolo*, ed. Ezio Riondato (Venice, 1985), pp. 1–28
——, *Fasciculo de medicina in volgare, Venezia, Giovanni e Gregorio De
    Gregori, 1494*, vol. I: *Facsimile dell'esemplare conservato presso la
    Biblioteca del Centro per la Storia dell'Università di Padova*; vol. II:
    Il 'Fasciculus medicinae' ovvero le metamorfosi del libro umanistico
    (Treviso, 2001)
Pormann, Peter E., and Emilie Savage-Smith, *Medieval Islamic Medicine*
    (Edinburgh, 2007)
Pouchelle, Marie-Christine, *The Body and Surgery in the Middle Ages*,
    trans. Rosemary Morris (Cambridge, 1990)
Premuda, Loris, *Storia dell'iconografia anatomica* (Milan, 1993)
Roberts, K. B., and J.D.W. Tomlinson, *The Fabric of the Body: European
    Traditions of Anatomical Illustration* (Oxford, 1992)

Robison, Kira, *Healers in the Making: Students, Physicians, and Medical Education in Medieval Bologna (1250–1550)* (Leiden and Boston, MA, 2021)

Rosenberg, Lauren, 'Image of Flesh/Flesh of the Image: the Flayed Figure in Henri de Mondeville's *Chirurgia*', *Object*, XX (2019), pp. 82–100

Savage-Smith, Emilie, 'Anatomical Illustration in Arabic Manuscripts', in *Arab Painting: Text and Image in Illustrated Arabic Manuscripts*, ed. Anna Contadini (Leiden, 2007)

Saxl, Fritz, 'A Spiritual Encyclopedia of the Later Middle Ages', *Journal of the Warburg and Courtauld Institutes*, V (1942), pp. 82–137

Schultz, Bernard, *Art and Anatomy in Renaissance Italy* (Ann Arbor, MI, 1985)

Seebohm, Almuth, *Apokalypse, ars moriendi, medizinische Traktate, Tugend- und Lasterlehren die erbaulich-didaktische Sammelhandschrift London, Wellcome Institute for the History of Medicine, Ms. 49: Farbmikrofiche-Edition* (Munich, 1994)

Singer, Charles, 'Note on a Thirteenth Century Diagram of the Male Genitalia', *Studies in the History and Method of Science*, I (1917), pp. 212–14

——, 'A Thirteenth Century Drawing of the Anatomy of the Uterus and Adnexa', *Studies in the History and Method of Science*, I (1917), pp. 43–7

——, 'Thirteenth-Century Miniatures Illustrating Medical Practice', *Proceedings of the Royal Society of Medicine*, IX (1915–16), pp. 29–41

Sudhoff, Karl, *Beiträge zur Geschichte der Chirurgie im Mittelalter, graphische und textliche Untersuchungen in mittelalterlichen Handschriften*, 2 vols (Leipzig, 1914–18)

——, *Ein Beitrag zur Geschichte der Anatomie im Mittelalter, speziell der anatomischen Graphik nach Handschriften des 9. bis 15. Jahrbunderts, Studien zur Geschichte der Medezin*, IV (Leipzig, 1908, repr. Hildesheim, 1964)

——, *Weitere Beiträge zur Geschichte der Anatomie im Mittelalter. Aus dem Institut für Geschichte der Medizin in Leipzig. IV. Archiv für Geschichte der Medizin*, VIII (Leipzig, 1914)

Svenberg, Torgny, and Peter Murray Jones, trans. and eds, *De Arte Phisicali et de Chirurgia by John Arderne; From a New Digital Version of the Stockholm Roll* (Stockholm, 2014)

Wallis, Faith, ed., *Medieval Medicine: A Reader* (Toronto, 2010)

Wickersheimer, Ernst, *Anatomies de Mondino de Liuzzi et de Guido de Vigevano* (Paris, 1926)

ACKNOWLEDGEMENTS

This book was made possible by a generous grant from the International Center of Medieval Art's Kress Publication Grant and research support from the Medieval Academy of America. I have benefited from the time and generosity of many scholars in the course of pursuing medieval anatomy. My deepest thanks go to Jack Hartnell and Adam Harris Levine for their diligent reading of this entire book, and to Peter Murray Jones and Monica H. Green for their constant willingness to consider various medical topics with me. I am especially grateful for Deirdre Jackson's keen editorial eye and insights, and to Michael Leaman, Phoebe Colley, Alex Ciobanu and the Reaktion team for their support and guidance in ushering this book to publication. The anonymous press reviewer prompted much reconsideration and reorganization, to great benefit. The seeds of this work were planted and nurtured during my time as a graduate and undergraduate researcher by the advice and critiques of Jean Michel Massing, Paul Binski, Alixe Bovey, John Lowden and Eric Ramírez-Weaver. Mary Carruthers, Teresa Webber, Christopher de Hamel and Peter Bovenmyer discussed specific manuscripts, images and scripts with me. I am also incredibly appreciative of the help offered by so many librarians and archivists as I trawled through their collections. This book would not have been possible without the efforts of collections staff members who so diligently and tirelessly produced online reproductions of their treasures. I thank my parents for their constant financial and moral support during my studies, my sister for always listening despite having no idea what I was talking about much of the time, and my friends and family for their love and enthusiasm during the decade I have been working on this subject. Finally, this is dedicated to John, whose perspective and encouragement has kept me going, and to Jack, whose arrival forced me to slow down and refocus, making life (and this book) infinitely richer.

PHOTO ACKNOWLEDGEMENTS

The author and publishers wish to express their thanks to the below sources of illustrative material and/or permission to reproduce it. Some locations of artworks are also given below, in the interest of brevity:

Bayerische Staatsbibliothek, Munich (CC BY-NC-SA 4.0): 2 (Clm 13002, fol. 2v), 3 (Clm 13002, fol. 3r), 15 (Clm 13002, fol. 7v); from Jacopo Berengario da Carpi, *Isagogae breves, perlucidae ac uberrimae, in anatomiam humani corporis* (Bologna, 1523), photo National Library of Medicine, Bethesda, MD: 62; Bibliothèque municipale de Besançon, photo © IRHT–CNRS (CC BY-NC 3.0): 7 (MS 457, fol. 248v); Bibliothèque municipale de Lyon, photo © IRHT–CNRS (CC BY-NC 3.0): 66 (Rés. Inc. 1042, fol. 44v); Bibliothèque du musée Condé, château de Chantilly, photos © IRHT–CNRS (CC BY-NC 3.0): 10 (MS 334, fol. 260v), 25 (MS 65, fol. 14v), 32 (MS 334, fol. 267v), 42 (MS 334, fol. 261r), 43 (MS 334, fol. 265v); Bibliothèque nationale de France, Paris: 6 (MS fr. 218, fol. 56r), 27 (MS fr. 134, fol. 48v), 35 (MS fr. 2030, fol. 29r), 52 (MS lat. 16169, fol. 59v), 53 (MS lat. 16169, fol. 176r), 68 (MS fr. 396, fol. 6v); Bibliothèque royale de Belgique, Brussels: 9 (MS 3701–15, fol. 27v); Bibliothèque universitaire de médecine, Montpellier, photo © IRHT–CNRS (CC BY-NC 3.0): 69 (MS H 184, fol. 14v); © Bodleian Libraries, University of Oxford (CC BY-NC 4.0): 20 (MS Ashmole 399, fol. 22r), 21 (MS Ashmole 399, fol. 23v), 22 (MS Ashmole 399, fol. 13v), 37 (MS Ashmole 399, fol. 34r); © The British Library Board: 36 (Sloane MS 1977, fol. 2v), 44 (Arundel MS 83, fol. 127r), 49 and 50 (Add. MS 8785, fol. 54r), 51 (Add. MS 8785, fol. 55v), 67 (Harley MS 4425, fol. 59r); from Mondino dei Liuzzi, *Anathomia* (Leipzig, c. 1493), photo Wellcome Collection, London (CC BY 4.0): 71; © The Fitzwilliam Museum, University of Cambridge: 28 (MS 167, fol. 102r); from Hans von Gersdorff, *Feldtbüch der Wundartzney* (Strasbourg, 1528), photos National Library of Medicine, Bethesda, MD: 11, 64; Gonville and Caius College, University of Cambridge, photos reproduced by permission of the Master and Fellows of Gonville and Caius College: 4 (MS 190/223, fol. 4v), 5 (MS 190/223, fol. 5r), 16 (MS 190/223, fol. 2v), 17 (MS 190/223, fol. 3r), 18 (MS 190/223, fol. 5v), 19 (MS 190/223, fol. 6r); from Johannes de Ketham, *Fasciculus medicinae* (Venice, 1491), photo Frances A. Countway Library of Medicine, Boston, MA: 33; from Johannes de Ketham, *Fasciculo de medicina*

INDEX OF MANUSCRIPTS CITED

Avignon, Bibliothèque
   municipale, MS 1019 135
Basel, Universitatsbibliothek,
   MS D II II 117, 120–23, *14, 47*
Besançon, Bibliothèque
   municipale, MS 457 136, *7*
Bethesda, MD, National Library of
   Medicine, MS P 18 117–23,
   12, 45, 46, 48
Brussels, Bibliothèque Royale,
   MS 3701–15 20, *9*
Cambridge
   Gonville and Caius College,
      MS 190/223 10, 42–50, *4, 5,
      16–19*
   Fitzwilliam Museum, MS 167
      70, *28*
   Trinity College, MS O.2.44
      102–4, *39, 40*
Chantilly, Bibliothèque du musée
   Condé
   MS 65 67–8, *25*
   MS 334 110–15, *10, 32, 42, 43*
Dessau-Rosslau, Landesbibliothek,
   MS Georg 271 71–3, *29*
El Escorial, Royal Library of the
   Monastery of El Escorial,
   MS T-I-I 96–7, *38*
Glasgow, University of Glasgow
   Library, MS Hunter 9
   167–9, *70*
London, British Library
   Additional MS 8785 130–32,
      49, 50, 51
   Arundel MS 83 113–14, *44*

   Harley MS 4425 163, *67*
   Sloane MS 1977 88, *36*
London, Wellcome Library
   MS 40 71, *26*
   MS 49 54, 57–60, 172, *23, 24,
      30, 31, 63*
   MS 290 142–3, 174, *59, 60,
      72*
   MS 349 70, *1*
Montpellier, Bibliothèque
   universitaire de médecine,
   MS H 184 166–7, *69*
Munich, Bayerische
   Staatsbibliothek
   Clm 13002 10, 20, 23, 32–6,
      40–41, 64–5 *2, 3, 15*
   Clm 13042 117
   Clm 17403 41–2
Oxford, Bodleian Library
   MS Ashmole 399 52–4, *20,
      21, 22, 37*
Paris, Bibliothèque nationale de
   France
   MS fr. 134 70, *27*
   MS fr. 218 160–62, *6*
   MS fr. 396 164–6, *68*
   MS fr. 2030 102–4, 127, *35*
   MS fr. 16169 132–5, *51, 52*
   MS fr. 22532 130
Philadelphia, PA, University of
   Pennsylvania, Rare Book and
   Manuscript Library, MS LJS
   24 130
Pisa, Biblioteca Universitaria,
   MS 735 52

Stockholm, National Library of Sweden,
    MS X 188   137–43, 54, 55, 56, 57
The Vatican, Biblioteca Apostolica
    Vaticana
    MS Pal. lat. 1110 117
    MSS Urb. lat. 240, 241 136

GENERAL INDEX

Illustration numbers are indicated by *italics*

Albertus Magnus 132–5, *52, 53*
Alderotti, Taddeo 92
Alhazen (Ḥasan ibn al-Haytham)
    18, 116, *8*
anatomical images
    and abstraction 43–50
    of the arteries *2, 16, 43*
    of the bones *3, 17, 23, 40, 45,*
        47, 54, 55, 59, 60, 61, 64,
    of the bladder 7, 11, 13, 14,
        43, 49, 52
    of the brain and eyes 8, 11,
        19, 45, 46, 47
    of the digestive system *1, 2, 5,*
        11, 12, 31, 39, 43, 48, 56,
        57, 63
    of the female reproductive
        system *18, 22, 24, 35, 51,*
        72
    of the gallbladder *5, 11, 13,*
        16, 21, 29, 52, 53, 56, 57, 63
    of the heart *1, 2, 5, 11, 12, 13,*
        16, 21, 29, 31, 33, 37, 38,
        43, 52, 53, 56, 57, 63, 72
    of the kidneys *5, 11, 13, 30,*
        31, 37, 43, 52, 53, 56, 57,
        63, 72
    of the liver *1, 2, 5, 11, 13, 14,*
        16, 21, 29, 37, 52, 53, 56,
        57, 63, 72
    of the lungs *37, 43, 48, 56,*
        57
    of the male reproductive
        system *4, 24, 50*
    of the muscles *3, 20, 62*
    of the nerves *3, 23, 46*
    of the spleen *2, 5, 11, 12, 13,*
        16, 21, 29, 43, 52, 53, 56, 57
    of the stomach *5, 7, 11, 21, 30,*
        35, 43, 52, 56, 57, 63, 72
    of the veins *2, 48, 63*
Aristotle 15–16, 133–4
Articella 51
autopsy 93–8, 163–7
    of holy women 96–7
    of women 94–8, *37, 38*
Avicenna (Ibn Sina) 129, 136,
    160
    Canon of Medicine 127, 129,
        136, 167–9, *7, 70*

Bartholomew the Englishman
    129–32
    *De proprietatibus rerum/Livre
        des propriétés des choses* 127,
        129–32, 160–63, 170, *6, 27,*
        49, 50, 51, 66
Benedict of Nursia 36–7
Berengario, Jacopo 149–51, *62*
bloodletting 66–7, 71–3, *26, 29*

Cantigas de Santa María 96–7, *38*
cautery 20, 33, 66, *2*
Chiara of Montefalco 96–7
Constantine the African 38–40,
    51
    Pantegni 39, 90, 92, 128–9
counterfeit 151–4, *11, 64*

Dance of Death 103, 142–3, 58
Disease Man 73
Disease Woman 73–80, 142–3,
   30, 33, 34, 72
dissection
   images of 6, 10, 41, 52, 53, 65,
      66, 68, 69, 70, 71
   in ancient medicine 15–17
   in Roman de la rose 163, 67
   in medical curricula 92,
      98–101

Fasciculus medicinae 80, 159,
   172–5, 33, 34, 65
Five-Figure Series 33–6, 41–3,
   57, 60, 71, 83, 102–3, 116,
   2, 3, 16, 17
foetus
   Muscio images see Muscio
   in full-body female figures 76,
      117, 30, 33, 48

Galen of Pergamum 15–17,
   39–40
Ghiberti, Lorenzo 146–7
Glossarium Salomonis 32
Gregori, Giovanni and Gregorio
   de 172
Guido of Vigevano 27, 29, 107–15,
   123–4, 176, 10, 32, 42–3
Guy of Chauliac 102, 160
   Chirurgia magna/La grande
      chirurgie 164–6, 68, 69
gynaecology 52–4, 76–80, 121–3
   and the bicornate uterus 46–7,
      9, 18, 22, 24
   and reproduction 46–7, 57,
      74–80, 123
   and the seven-celled uterus 76,
      99–100, 113, 115, 123, 132
      14, 32

Hagenauer, Nikolaus 154
Henry of Mondeville 83–6, 101–5,
   123–4, 35, 40
herbal 20
Herophilus and Erasistratus 17
Heymandus de Veteri Busco 70, 1
Hippocrates 15–16
Historia incisionis 34, 39–43, 52,
   91, 99
Hock, Wendelin 151–4, 11
humoral theory 15, 63
Hutz, Mathieu 161–2

Johannes Grusch atelier 135–6, 7
John of Arderne 137–42

Lanfranc of Milan 90–91, 111
Leonardo da Vinci 23, 148–9, 13
Limbourg Brothers 67–8, 25

Mansūr ibn Muḥammad ibn
   Amād ibn Yūsuf ibn Ilyās
   29, 116–17
   Tashrīḥ-i Manṣūr-i 116–23,
      12, 45, 46, 48
Margarita of Città di Castello 96
Masaccio 147, 61
melothesia see zodiac
Michelangelo 149
microcosm 63–6, 15
Mondino dei Liuzzi 86, 98–101
   Anathomia 98–101, 111,
      170, 176, 65, 71
Montpellier, University of 91, 100
Muscio 20
   foetal images associated with
      20, 137, 9, 24
Nine-Figure Series 43–50, 52–60,
   99, 111, 126, 158
Notke, Berndt (workshop of)
   142–3, 58

phlebotomy *see* bloodletting
planetary figure 70, *28*
post-mortem *see* autopsy
Prüfening, Benedictine
     abbey of 32–4, 40–41

Raphael 149
rational surgeons 90–91
Roger Frugardi 88, *36*

Salernitan Demonstrations,
     the 92–3
Salerno
     medical teaching at 50–51, 86,
        92–3
     Trota of 94
Scheyern, Benedictine monastery
     of 41–2
Schott, Johannes 151, *11*
surgery
     and anatomy 90–91
     in universities 86–9
Syber, Jean 160–62, *66*

Tacuinum sanitatis 71–2
Three-Figure Series 73
Three Living and the Three Dead
     113–14, *44*

University of Bologna 86, 91–2,
     100
University of Paris 51, 88, 91, 127
urinoscopy 38–9

Vesalius, Andreas 29, 106–7,
     158–60, 175–6, *41*

William of Saliceto 90
Wound Man 73, *31*

zodiac 66–71, *1*, *25*, *27*